FORENSICS

FORENSICS

The Science Behind the
Deaths of Famous People

HARRY A. MILMAN, PHD

To order additional copies of this book, contact:
Xlibris
844-714-8691
www.Xlibris.com
Orders@Xlibris.com
810738

To indie authors everywhere

CONTENTS

ACKNOWLEDGMENTS

A SPECIAL THANK you to Caren Milman, whose careful editing and helpful suggestions made this book possible.

My sincere gratitude to Teri Hawn, Jeffrey Hyman, and Robert Emery, who provided critical and thoughtful insight and direction in the early phases of the manuscript.

Thank you to Jennifer McGinn of Jennifer McGinn Photography for her excellent photographic skills, especially during the COVID-19 pandemic. You're the best!

Thank you to Elizabeth of the editorial staff of Xlibris for her excellent line editing and to Joe Scaggs for his commitment to excellence in the publication of all three of my books.

I am indebted to Barnes & Noble Booksellers and its nationwide staff who hosted me for more than 175 book-signing events since 2015.

And lastly, my heartfelt thanks to all my fans who supported me throughout the tortuous road to success.

INTRODUCTION

IN 1888, PUBLIC fascination with criminal investigations was at an all-time high, mainly because of two highly publicized events. Jack the Ripper was murdering prostitutes and mutilating their bodies in areas in and around the Whitechapel district of London, and Sir Arthur Conan Doyle, the British author, published his Sherlock Holmes novels. Doyle's books featured a private detective who used logic and forensic science, the application of scientific principles and methods to civil and criminal laws, to help solve crimes. Today, interest in forensics, especially among young people, continues to remain strong, mostly due to crime recreation television shows, as well as programs such as *CSI: Crime Scene Investigation*, *Bones*, and *Cold Case*.[1] These fictionalized portrayals of the daily work of forensic scientists have glamorized the profession, so much so that the so-called CSI effect has led to an explosion of high school, undergraduate, and graduate programs that specialize in various subspecialties of forensic science, including forensic toxicology.[1] Equally important, there is a newly heightened public awareness in criminal investigations and the importance of securing a crime scene, how to avoid contaminating key evidence, and the power and limitations of laboratory tests.

Forensics in Crime Investigation

The use of forensics in a murder investigation can be traced back to 44 BC when the first officially recorded autopsy was conducted by Antistius, a Roman physician.[2] The autopsy was performed on the body of Gaius Julius Caesar, a decorated general and one of the most powerful and influential Roman politicians, whose death was forever immortalized by William Shakespeare in his historical play *The Tragedy of Julius Caesar*.[3] Antistius identified twenty-three stab wounds, including some on Caesar's face and groin, with the fatal blow entering Caesar's body just beneath his left shoulder blade at an angle that struck his heart and possibly the aorta, the largest artery in the body.[3] Death occurred slowly as a result of Caesar's substantial internal bleeding and collapsed lungs.[3] When Antistius presented his findings to the Roman people, he became the first medical doctor to act as an expert witness in a murder inquiry.[3]

Xi Yuan Lu, translated as *Washing Away of Wrongs,* was the first treatise to describe the use of medicine and entomology, the scientific study of insects, to distinguish between suicide, murder, and an accidental death.[4] Written by Song Ci during the Song dynasty, *Xi Yuan Lu* was published in China in the thirteenth century.

Henry Goddard of London's Scotland Yard launched the field of forensic ballistics in 1835 when he connected a bullet to a murder weapon.[5] This new subspecialty of forensic science was further advanced in the late 1970s when a method was developed that used an electron microscope to detect gunshot residues.[5]

A classification system for analyzing fingerprints was created in 1896 by Sir Edward Richard Henry, London's commissioner of the Metropolitan Police. Using the direction, flow, pattern, and other characteristics in fingerprints, suspects in crimes were now able to be more easily identified.[5] Edmond Locard, known as the "Sherlock Holmes of France," improved the science of fingerprint analysis further when he discovered that a positive identification of an individual could be made if twelve specific points were identical between two fingerprints.[6] Locard's discovery was instrumental in helping police investigators to apprehend criminals. The Federal Bureau of Investigation, or FBI, has since modified the so-called Henry Classification System, making it the gold standard of criminal fingerprint analysis.[7]

Modern-Day Forensics

Modern-day forensics is a scientific tool that helps identify and evaluate evidence in support of criminal and civil legal investigations. One of the most important scientific concepts that formed the basis of modern-day forensics was provided by Locard, the same French physician and criminologist who improved the science of fingerprint analysis.[8]

Locard had a strong interest in forensic science and had worked as a medical examiner with the French Secret Service during World War I.[8] He was the first to establish a police crime laboratory in Lyon, France, in 1910.[8] Locard's exchange principle, a theory Locard proposed in his seven-volume series, *Treaty of Criminalistics*, forever changed the way crime investigations were conducted.[8] It stated, "It is impossible for a criminal to act, considering the intensity of the crime, without leaving a trace."[9] Thus, trace evidence, no matter how infinitesimal, told a story that could be helpful in a crime scene investigation.[10] It's due to Locard's exchange principle that DNA analysis, first applied in 1985 in a double-murder case in a small town in England, as well as DNA profiling have led to the successful identification of criminals, while at the same time exonerating prisoners for crimes they did not commit.[11]

Forensic Toxicology

In the nineteenth century, arsenic, which has a sweet taste and could be mixed with food, was being used in poisonings because it left no visible signs of foul play and was untraceable in the body.[12] Criminal investigations of arsenic poisonings were significantly improved when toxicology, the study of poisons, was introduced and quickly became recognized as an important forensic investigative tool.

Carl Wilhelm Scheele, a Swedish chemist and pharmacist who discovered oxygen and other elements, was studying methods for measuring arsenic in humans. He noticed that when arsenic oxide was chemically reacted with zinc and nitric acid, a gas with a distinctive garlic smell was formed.[13] Using his new methodology, Scheele was able to detect high concentrations of arsenic in a corpse.[14] Valentin Ross, a German chemist, expanded on Scheele's work, and in 1806, he developed a method for detecting arsenic in the walls of a victim's stomach.[15] Thirty years later, the Scottish chemist James Marsh was the first to apply the scientific methods of arsenic detection to a murder trial.[16] His Marsh test—a chemical reaction between arsenic, zinc, and sulfuric acid that could measure as little as twenty micrograms of arsenic—is still being used today.[17]

The field of forensic toxicology was further enriched by the work of Karl Landsteiner on blood groups.[18] Born in Vienna, Austria, Landsteiner's interests in morbid anatomy, morbid physiology, and immunology eventually brought him to the Rockefeller Institute for Medical Research in New York.[18] His classification of blood into four separate types, A, B, AB, and O, for which Landsteiner was awarded the Nobel Prize in Physiology or Medicine in 1930, was a major breakthrough for forensic toxicologists and police investigators, as it provided significant leads to help solve crimes.[18]

Since poisons must enter blood before they can exert their toxic effects, forensic toxicologists employ scientific principles dealing with absorption, distribution, metabolism, and elimination to determine the harmful effects caused by drugs and toxic chemicals.[19] By the mid-1990s, several methods had been developed that could detect poisons not only in blood but in various other bodily fluids as well, such as saliva, semen, sweat, and urine.[20]

Working in forensic laboratories, forensic toxicologists conduct physical and chemical tests on evidence obtained at crime scenes, acquired at autopsies, or obtained during drug monitoring. They utilize various analytical techniques, the most common of which are immunoassays using antibody reactions, to detect toxicants in bodily fluids.[21] However, these screening tests do not quantify and are subject to false-positive and false-negative results. Any presumptive positive must first be verified by a second confirmatory test before it can be applied in decision-making. These highly specific confirmatory techniques often combine gas chromatography and mass spectrometry methodologies. Unlike immunoassay screens, they can detect as well as quantify the amount of a substance in a biological sample.[21]

Blood is the specimen of choice to establish whether human performance or behavior, as in driving, has been impaired by drugs or alcohol or whether a drug overdose has caused death.[21] However, urine is the biological fluid most commonly examined during random drug testing in the workplace, as well as to control doping in sports and to monitor compliance with probation and parole.[21] Unlike with blood, positive results in a urine test do not correlate with drug effects at the time of sampling. They merely identify drugs being eliminated from the body. Similarly, a positive finding of drugs in the liver, where metabolism occurs, or in the vitreous humor, the gel-like substance in the eye, indicates that the drugs had been consumed sometime prior to sampling. However, when a positive finding is obtained in a hair specimen, which is subject to contamination, or in fingernail or toenail clippings, it indicates that a drug had been consumed weeks or possibly even months before the sample was tested.

In postmortem forensic investigations, forensic pathologists and medical examiners perform autopsies and identify anatomical abnormalities that may be related to cause of death. Any blood, urine, or tissue specimens collected at the autopsy are then examined by forensic toxicologists who identify and quantify any toxicants present in the samples.[21] Results obtained from tests performed using postmortem blood, or blood taken after death, could be difficult to interpret since postmortem redistribution may have taken place. This is a time during which the blood concentration of a drug could rise, sometimes by as much as two- to threefold, as reequilibration occurs from sites of higher drug concentration, such as the lungs, liver, and heart, into blood.[22] Nevertheless, after reviewing the autopsy findings and toxicology test results, coroners then provide a medical opinion, within the guidelines prescribed in the *Physicians' Handbook on Medical Certification of Death* of the US Centers for Disease Control and Prevention, on the likely cause and manner of death.[23]

While forensics provides a scientific explanation for an injury or a disease that could then be used to determine cause of death, manner of death, for which there are five possible categories—natural, accident, suicide, homicide, and undetermined—is a medicolegal interpretation of the circumstances that led to a death. When manner of death is in dispute, it can lead to conspiracy theories.

In addition to their other activities, forensic toxicologists and other discipline-specific forensic experts often provide expert testimony at trials and depositions. Before they can testify, however, they must first pass the Daubert standard.[24] Based on a 1993 Supreme Court case, *Daubert v. Merrell Dow Pharmaceuticals, Inc.,* a trial judge assesses whether an expert witness's testimony will be scientifically valid before he allows the expert to testify at trial. In federal and most state courts, Daubert has replaced the Frye standard that was established in 1923 in *Frye v. United States.*[25]

As a PhD pharmacologist and toxicologist with substantial experience reviewing medical and autopsy records, toxicology reports and the scientific literature, I have assisted in more than three hundred civil, criminal, and high-profile cases and have provided expert testimony at trials and depositions. In this book, I investigated the deaths of twenty-three famous people based on a review of publicly available autopsy and toxicology reports, as well as published scientific and lay articles. My aim was to demonstrate how forensics helps coroners determine that 51 percent or more of the evidence supports an opinion that death more likely than not was caused by drugs, chemical toxicants, or disease, the standard by which expert testimony is judged in court.

CHAPTER 1

Errol Flynn

Died October 14, 1959

BY MID-1940, ERROL Flynn, an actor who portrayed swashbuckling characters on the big screen, was rich, famous, and a bachelor, having divorced his wife, an actress five years his senior.[1] "Women won't let me stay single, and I won't let myself stay married," he said at the time.[2] However, by the late 1950s, his best days were behind him.[2] His career was in a steep decline, and his playboy lifestyle had aged him prematurely. With little income, two divorces, and a penchant for drinking alcohol that had dramatically escalated, reportedly to about two to three quarts of vodka a day, Flynn's personal fortune was nearly depleted.[2] To raise money so he could divorce his third wife and marry his seventeen-year-old girlfriend, Beverly Aadland, Flynn had to sell or lease his only remaining significant asset, his yacht, the *Zacca*.[3] People often raised their eyebrows at the sight of his latest flame, but Flynn didn't care. "I like my whiskey old and my women young," he would tell them in no uncertain terms.[4]

Sometime in early October 1959, Flynn called his old friend George Caldough, a prominent stockbroker in Vancouver, Canada, to ask if he was still interested in purchasing his yacht.[5] Caldough said he was and arranged to meet Flynn in Hollywood the following week.[5] "We hadn't met in two years, but he had aged twenty," Caldough later recalled.[5] Ten days after they reconnected in California, Flynn and Aadland followed Caldough to West Vancouver.[5]

Flynn planned to return to the United States on October 14; however, he had been suffering from intermittent low back and leg pain for several months, especially during the last two days before his departure from Vancouver.[6] Caldough suggested they stop to see his friend Dr. Grant Gould on the way to the airport so Flynn could receive something for his pain.[6] Gould had just completed his office hours and told Caldough that they should come to his house instead.[6] By the time they arrived at Gould's residence, Flynn wasn't able to flex his left leg without experiencing excruciating pain and had to be helped up the stairs.[6]

After examining Flynn, Gould diagnosed him with "acute intervertebral disc syndrome with sciatica radiation, producing intense muscle spasm and pain down the left leg and in the lower back."[6] Flynn, who was in pain every time he sat down, remained standing while Gould treated him with an intravenous injection of a therapeutic dose of meperidine, an opioid analgesic medication.[6] The drug must have taken effect very quickly because almost as soon as it was injected, Flynn said he felt "ever so much better."[6] However, before he attempted to walk again, Gould had Flynn lie down on the bedroom floor so he could massage his left leg, which provided Flynn additional relief from his pain.[6]

At 6:45 p.m., about twenty minutes after Gould administered the intravenous injection, Aadland came running out of the bedroom saying Flynn had suddenly collapsed, his color was poor, and he had stopped breathing.[6] Gould rushed to Flynn's aid and listened for a heartbeat, but it was very faint.[6] He immediately injected epinephrine, a lifesaving hormone that stimulates the heart, directly into Flynn's heart.[6] At the same time, he instructed Aadland to give Flynn mouth-to-mouth resuscitation, which she promptly did.[6] Surprisingly, she then pulled a box of amyl nitrite ampules from her purse and quickly broke one under Flynn's nose.[6] The drug is used to treat angina, chest pain caused by reduced blood flow to the heart. "This was the first indication [I had] of any previous cardiac involvement," Gould would later write to Glen McDonald, the coroner of the city of Vancouver.[6] Unlike most, if not all, coroners who are physicians, McDonald was a lawyer and a judge, not a medical doctor.[7]

Paramedics arrived within minutes and administered oxygen to Flynn.[8] Flynn still wasn't responding to the treatment by 7:15, so they transferred him to Vancouver General Hospital, where he was pronounced dead a half an hour later.[8] He was fifty years old.

The Autopsy

Flynn's autopsy was performed by Dr. T. R. Harmon on October 15, 1959.[8] "This is the body of a well-nourished, well-developed, white male, seventy-three and a half inches in length and weighing approximately two-hundred and twenty-five pounds," Harmon wrote in the autopsy report.[8] His description of Flynn's body was deceptive, however, because severe, life-threatening anatomical abnormalities became apparent as soon as the internal organs were revealed.[8]

The presence of "condyloma acuminata" or genital warts, a sexually transmitted infection on Flynn's penis caused by the human papillomavirus, corroborated Flynn's reputation for numerous sexual liaisons.[9] "All over the world I was, as a name and personality, equated with sex," he once said.[10] Other findings observed upon external examination included superficial scars and crusted, scaled, uninflamed areas on both of Flynn's legs as well as scars on both of his knees.[11]

The circumstances surrounding Flynn's death strongly suggested he had suffered a heart-related event, so I was especially interested to review the autopsy findings of his cardiovascular system. A close examination of the heart showed evidence of an acute infarction—recent death of heart muscle caused by obstruction of the blood supply to the left ventricle, one of the heart chambers.[11] It was accompanied by marked pallor or paleness and mottled appearance of the heart muscle, both of which were due to the poor blood supply to the heart.[11] In addition, there was evidence of atherosclerosis, a marked accumulation of large plaques in and narrowing of the coronary arteries and aorta (the main artery that supplies oxygenated blood to the rest of the body), as well as a recent blood clot that plugged the lumen of one of the coronary arteries.[11] All of these cardiovascular findings were consistent with Flynn having recently suffered a heart attack.[11] Furthermore, at nearly twice its normal weight, Flynn's heart was a risk factor for sudden death from an arrhythmia, an electrical abnormality in the heart that causes an irregular heartbeat and could lead to death.[11]

Flynn's cardiac anomalies weren't his only medical problem. His liver was pale and had a yellowish-tan or brownish-tan color, and its surface was finely nodular in some areas, unlike a normal liver that is reddish brown and smooth.[11] Furthermore, Flynn's liver weighed more than twice the average weight of a normal liver.[12] And when it was sliced, there was some resistance, suggesting the presence of moderate portal cirrhosis, a chronic liver disease typically caused by alcoholism.[12] This was confirmed when samples of liver tissue were examined under a microscope and showed evidence of early portal cirrhosis, as well as fatty metamorphosis, a condition often seen in alcoholics in which excess fat is stored in the liver.[13]

Flynn's remaining organs—the lungs, spleen, and kidneys—were markedly congested, possibly indicative of cardiovascular disease or heart failure, with a large amount of mucus in the lungs and blood clots in some of the lung arteries. Also, diverticulae or "pockets" were apparent in the walls of the colon as well as marked osteoarthritis in the spine.[13] None of these findings, however, were the cause of Flynn's death.

While malaria parasites were not detected in Flynn's spleen, laboratory tests identified an increased number of eosinophils, a type of disease-fighting white blood cell, probably due to Flynn's recurring bouts with malaria from when he was in New Guinea.[13]

After reviewing the autopsy findings, I had no doubt Flynn was in very poor health prior to his death. His liver was barely functional, his lungs, kidneys, and spleen were markedly congested, and his severely atherosclerotic and mottled heart was ready to explode with a massive heart attack at a moment's notice. According to one report, Flynn's body was likened to a seventy-five-year-old man.[14] The coroner, however, described it as more like an eighty-five-year-old man.[14] Whatever the age, of one thing I was certain: Flynn's heart, liver, and penis had taken their share of abuse from his long-term, excessive consumption of alcohol and indiscriminate sexual dalliances.

Cause and Manner of Death

Gould, the same physician who treated Flynn's back and leg pain, concluded Flynn died as "a result of a sudden, overwhelming myocardial infarction [heart attack] of such proportions as to produce death without premonitory symptoms."[15] According to McDonald, the coroner, an investigation by the Vancouver City Police Department found no evidence of violence or any suspicion of foul play.[15] While McDonald acknowledged the autopsy findings related to the cardiovascular system and liver, he labeled Flynn's manner of death as due to natural causes.[15] However, considering Flynn had these life-threatening anatomical abnormalities for many weeks and possibly even months, the question I was left with after I reviewed the autopsy findings was, What led him to die on that particular day?

I had hoped to examine the toxicology report, but unfortunately, it wasn't available for review. Nevertheless, McDonald noted that the toxicology examination was exhaustive and did not disclose any "poison or foreign substance which could be directly associated in any way with [Flynn's] death."[15] However, he did mention that Flynn's blood alcohol concentration was at more than three times the current legal limit for drivers in the United States.[15] That amount of alcohol, McDonald decided, "would appear not to have been unusual for the deceased to have been able to handle without difficulty."[15] In addition, "the fact that no Demerol [meperidine] was found toxicologically would appear to confirm that the dosage given by Dr. Grant A. Gould was therapeutic," McDonald concluded.[15]

It's impossible to verify whether Flynn's blood was free of meperidine as McDonald claimed. However, the drug has a half-life, the time for half the concentration of the drug to be eliminated from the blood, of three hours in healthy people and more than six hours in people with cirrhosis of the liver.[16] Since Flynn had suffered from cirrhosis of the liver and he died only twenty minutes after Gould administered the opioid, meperidine should have been detected in his blood, unless the methodology for measuring the drug wasn't as sensitive then as it is today.[17]

It's unlikely Flynn's death was caused by the combined central nervous system depressant and sedative effects of meperidine and alcohol. While sedation is much more severe when the two drugs are taken together, there is no evidence Flynn was sedated, unconscious, or in a coma shortly before he died or that he suffered from respiratory depression. In addition, I have no reason to suspect Gould administered Flynn an opioid overdose.

Several scientific studies have shown that when meperidine is given intravenously, it can cause electrical abnormalities in the heart, such as QT elongation, a change that is readily seen on an electrocardiogram, as well as various types of arrhythmia, both of which could have caused Flynn's death.[18] Studies have further shown that when an intravenous injection of meperidine is given too quickly, it can produce a drop in blood pressure or hypotension, a slowing of the heart rate known as bradycardia, and even cardiac arrest or stoppage of the heart, any one of which could have caused Flynn to die. [19] Taken together, along with Flynn's significant risk factors for a cardiac-related event—an enlarged heart and severe coronary atherosclerosis—and the rapid onset of Flynn's cardiac arrest following the administration of meperidine, it's likely that Flynn's death may have been expedited by his treatment with meperidine. If so, his death was an accident, not natural. Further, had Flynn not been treated with meperidine, he may have remained alive to see another day, although it's impossible to predict how much longer he would have lived.

Life and Career

Born in 1909 in Tasmania, Australia, Flynn's childhood was an unhappy one, suffering physical and mental abuse by his mother.[20] When he was fourteen years old, he was sent to a boarding school in south London for two years. [21] This was followed by attendance at a boarding school in Sydney, Australia, from which he was expelled for fighting.[21] At eighteen, he ran away to New Guinea, where he worked as a guide, a plantation overseer, and a gold miner.[22] After several years, he returned to Australia, and much to his surprise, he was given the role of Fletcher Christian in the 1933 film *In the Wake of the Bounty.*[22] The movie wasn't a success at the box office, but it inspired Flynn, who had never considered a career in film, to become very interested in acting.

In late 1933, Flynn traveled to England, where he appeared in *Murder at Monte Carlo.*[22] Impressed with his performance, a talent scout for Warner Brothers cast Flynn in two minor films in the United States.[22] Later, when Robert Donat, an actor who was best known for his performances in *The 39 Steps* and *Goodbye, Mr. Chips,* turned down a role in the pirate epic *Captain Blood,* Flynn was selected to play the lead opposite the nineteen-year-old Olivia de Havilland.[22] The film became a huge success and catapulted Flynn to superstardom.[22] Over the course of his career, Flynn and de Havilland made eight movies together.[23] "Yes, we did fall in love and I believe that this is evident in the screen chemistry between us," de Havilland said in a 2009 interview when she was ninety-two years old.[24] "I have not talked about it a great deal, but the relationship was not consummated."[24]

Flynn appeared in several top-grossing films in the late 1930s to early 1940s, including *The Charge of the Light Brigade* (1936), *The Dawn Patrol* (1938), *The Adventures of Robin Hood* (1938), arguably his most famous and most enduring film, and *The Sea Hawk* (1940).[25] An exceptionally handsome, tall, and athletic actor with an on-screen charisma and a pencil mustache, Flynn became one of Warner Brothers' top stars during Hollywood's Golden Age.[26] Dashing, flamboyant, and charming in both his personal life and in his professional career, Flynn's movies earned millions of dollars, and he lived in the fast lane. Always with a beautiful woman on his arm and an alcoholic drink in his hand, Flynn not only starred as Don Juan, he was Don Juan.

Flynn's career began to unravel in November 1942, after he was indicted on three rape charges involving girls under the age of eighteen.[27] Although he was acquitted of all charges, the public's perception of Flynn began to change.[27] Despite becoming an American citizen, Flynn's image was further damaged when he received an 4-F deferment during World War II for health reasons—a heart murmur, bouts of malaria, which he had contracted in New Guinea, and latent tuberculosis.[28] In addition, his playboy lifestyle finally caught up with him in a dramatic way. His chronic, excessive drinking led Flynn to develop cirrhosis of the liver, and he contracted genital warts as a result of his many sexual exploits. Reportedly smoking one pack a day, Flynn's nicotine habit undoubtedly contributed to his cardiovascular disease and at least one and possibly two heart attacks.

FORENSICS

[28] When he was warned to take better care of himself, Flynn replied, "I intend to live the first half of my life. I don't care about the rest."[28] He got his wish.

Thankfully, the public was left with a treasure trove of Flynn's adventure movies, many of which can still be viewed today. Of these, the most celebrated is *The Adventures of Robin Hood*, in which Flynn played the legendary outlaw who "stole from the rich and gave to the poor." His performance in the film would forever link his name with Robin Hood.

Conclusion

Although the official cause of Flynn's death was a heart attack caused by a blockage of the coronary arteries, there is some evidence to suggest it may have been facilitated by his treatment with meperidine. In today's times, I could easily see this as grounds for litigation in a medical malpractice suit. Many similar cases have been litigated with much less scientific support. However, be that as it may, if there is one lesson that should be learned from Flynn's death, it is that abuse of one's body can lead to significant health consequences, whether by consuming an excessive amount of alcohol, ingesting large amounts of pharmaceuticals, or by experimenting with illicit drugs.

CHAPTER 2

Marilyn Monroe
Died August 4, 1962

ON AUGUST 4, 1962, Marilyn Monroe, a thirty-six-year-old actress who many thought was the sexiest woman in the world, was home in the Brentwood neighborhood of Los Angeles, speaking with her publicist in the morning, seeing her psychiatrist, Dr. Ralph Greenson, in the late afternoon, until about seven in the evening, and making phone calls late into the night.[1] Her housekeeper had stayed overnight but awoke at about three in the morning.[2] When she saw a light coming from under Monroe's bedroom door, she tried the door, but it was locked, so she called out for Monroe by name, but she received no reply.[2] Immediately, she telephoned Greenson, who broke one of the bedroom windows and entered the room.[2]

Greenson found Monroe lying on the bed with her phone in one hand and several prescription vials on her nightstand.[3] One of the vials was for pentobarbital, a barbiturate and sedative prescribed to help her sleep.[4] It was completely empty. Another was a partially empty bottle of chloral hydrate, also known as "Mickie Finn," a potent sedative and hypnotic medication.[5]

Monroe's personal physician was summoned at 4:25 a.m. and pronounced Monroe dead.[6] He estimated the time of death at sometime between eight thirty and ten thirty the previous evening, only three months after Monroe sang in front of fifteen thousand spectators for the president of the United States.[7]

The public was understandably curious to know how Monroe died. Everyone had a theory. Some believed she was murdered by the president of the United States and his brother, the attorney general, or possibly by the Mafia or even by the CIA. Others thought her death was a suicide committed by a lonely and insecure woman who was unable to cope with the demands of the film industry. Still others wondered whether it was an unfortunate accident that had gone awry. It was a question I was determined to investigate and whose answer I hoped to put to rest, once and for all.

The Autopsy

Monroe's autopsy was conducted at ten thirty on the morning of August 5, 1962, by Dr. Thomas T. Noguchi, a deputy medical examiner of the county of Los Angeles. [8] Born in Fukuoka, Japan, Noguchi studied medicine at the Nippon Medical School in Tokyo.[9] After a one-year internship, he immigrated to California, where he joined the medical examiner-coroner office.[9]

Noguchi was keenly aware that numerous conspiracy theories would emerge after he issued his final report, so he made sure the autopsy was thorough and complete. Slowly and methodically, he went about his work, pulling away the sheet and exposing the upper part of the body. "The unembalmed body is that of a thirty-six year old well-developed Caucasian female weighing one hundred and seventeen pounds and measuring sixty-five and a half inches in length," he wrote in his report.[10] "The scalp is covered with bleached blond hair. The eyes are blue."

From the outset, it seemed unlikely foul play was involved in Monroe's death. Her body had no gunshot wounds, punctures of the skin, or stab wounds, and it was found alone in Monroe's bedroom with the door locked from the inside.[11] Also, there were no skull fractures or trauma to the extremities, the neck, the scalp, or the forehead.[12] And when Noguchi examined the brain, he didn't find any gross abnormalities, contusions, or hemorrhage to suggest Monroe was hit on the head or had suffered a concussion, as from a fall.[12]

The stomach exhibited marked congestion with "petechial mucosal hemorrhage."[12] These lesions are commonly seen at autopsy and may be a side effect of some medications.[12] In addition, the colon was congested and had some purple discoloration, possibly from the use of laxatives.[12]

Since heart disease, which can also occur in young people, is the number one cause of death in the United States, I was especially interested in the autopsy findings related to Monroe's cardiovascular system. I first reviewed the size of the heart, because had it been enlarged, it would have been a risk factor for sudden death, but it was of normal size and weight.[12] Next, I looked for anatomical defects in the heart that might have led to a heart attack, but there weren't any.[12] Everything about the cardiovascular system appeared normal. The membranes surrounding the heart were smooth and glistening, the muscles in two of the four heart chambers were of normal size, the heart strings were not thickened or shortened, the heart valves between the heart chambers had the usual number of leaflets and were pliable, and the partitions separating the heart chambers were without defect.[12] Also, the arteries leading from the heart were normal, and there was no evidence of a clot in the artery leading to the lungs.[12] Had there been one, it could have impeded blood flow and might have led to a stroke or possibly even death.

Some published reports claimed Monroe drank too much alcohol, but if that was true, it wasn't reflected in the autopsy. People who drink alcohol to excess over many years often suffer from fatty metamorphosis or "fatty liver," a condition seen in Errol Flynn. However, Monroe's liver was smooth with no evidence of a hemorrhage or a tumor, and its weight was in the normal range.[12] Also, no alcohol was detected in Monroe's blood.[12]

The autopsy did reveal some interesting findings that were unrelated to cause of death.[12] For example, there was a three-inch horizontal surgical scar on the right upper quadrant of Monroe's abdomen consistent with past surgeries to remove her gallbladder and appendix, both of which were absent.[12] Also, a surgical scar identified above her pubic area measured five inches in length and may have been from a past surgery for an ectopic pregnancy, when Monroe was married to Arthur Miller, the playwright.[12] And while Monroe's lungs were moderately congested, there was only an insignificant amount of edema—fluid in the lungs.[12] Lastly, when Noguchi examined the body with a magnifying glass, he didn't find any needle marks.[12] This convinced me that Monroe's death wasn't caused by an injection of a drug overdose.

After completing my review of the autopsy report, I wasn't any closer to understanding how or why Monroe died, but of one thing I was certain. It wasn't because of a heart-related event such as an arrhythmia, or from a heart attack—death of heart muscle caused by blockage of the coronary arteries. Monroe was a young woman with a normally functioning heart, and her arteries and lungs were free of clots. And while her lungs were moderately congested, there was no evidence of bronchopneumonia, a respiratory problem that potentially could cause death. [12] However, since the autopsy only looked for anatomical changes, none of which were significant, I was anxious to review the toxicology report, hoping it would provide the necessary clues to help explain why Monroe died.

Cause and Manner of Death

It was well known that Monroe had attempted suicide on more than one occasion by swallowing a large amount of sleeping pills. [13] Since an empty bottle of pentobarbital was found by her bedside and forty capsules of chloral hydrate were missing from her prescription vial, I thought she might have done so again. My suspicion was confirmed when I reviewed the toxicology report and saw that pentobarbital was detected in blood taken at Monroe's autopsy. Its concentration was one and a half times more than the amount previously reported in people who had died from a pentobarbital overdose. [14] Also found in Monroe's blood was a large amount of chloral hydrate. [15] Both drugs depress the central nervous system and cause drowsiness when taken alone at therapeutic doses. However, when taken together at the high levels measured in Monroe's blood, their combined effect could be deadly. [16]

Conspiracy theorists pointed to the absence of yellow dye from the pentobarbital pills and the lack of pill residues in the stomach as evidence Monroe didn't take the barbiturate orally. The drug must have been administered by someone else, they claimed, if not by injection then in the form of a suppository. However, Noguchi didn't find any needle marks on Monroe's body. And since the stomach was almost completely empty, Monroe must have swallowed the drug on an empty stomach, a time when absorption is most rapid. It explained why there were no pill residues or dye in Monroe's stomach.

Having reviewed the toxicology report, I was now convinced Monroe died from acute barbiturate poisoning. [17] The amount of pentobarbital in her blood was over the lethal limit, and chloral hydrate was also very high. She would have had to swallow many pills to achieve those levels, so most likely, she had done so by herself and was not force-fed the medications.[17]

Invariably, Monroe's death spiral began with drowsiness, but it was quickly followed by marked sedation, slowed and shallow breathing, an inability to provide sufficient oxygen to the brain, a drop in blood pressure followed by circulatory collapse, as well as respiratory depression, coma, and ultimately death. It explained why several of Monroe's friends reported that on the night she died, Monroe's speech was slurred, most likely from oversedation, and she sounded as if she was under the influence of drugs.[18] It also explained why Monroe's body was found lying on the bed and why her housekeeper didn't hear anything unusual coming from Monroe's bedroom. A question still remained to be answered, however: was Monroe's death intentional or an unfortunate accident?

Dr. Thomas J. Curphey, the reform-minded pathologist and chief medical examiner-coroner, was reluctant to classify Monroe's death a suicide without a suicide note. To assist him with a "psychological autopsy," something that had never been done before, he recruited a team of top-notch psychiatrists with impeccable credentials whose opinions would not be challenged.[19] He hoped the psychiatric team would provide its expert opinion regarding Monroe's intent at the time she ingested the sedative drugs that ultimately led to her death.[19]

After painstakingly reviewing all the relevant records, the psychiatric investigative team concluded that since Monroe had been taking sedative drugs for many years, she should have been well aware of their dangers. Further, on more than one occasion, when she was disappointed and depressed, she had attempted suicide using sedative drugs but had called for help and had been rescued in time. However, on the night of August 4–5, 1962, she did so again, but unfortunately the outcome was different. [19] The large amount of barbiturate and chloral hydrate in Monroe's blood, the empty pentobarbital bottle, and the missing chloral hydrate capsules, as well as the locked door to Monroe's bedroom all led the team of psychiatrists to recommend that the manner of Monroe's death should be classified a probable suicide.[19]

On August 18, 1962, Curphey delivered his final opinion on the cause and manner of Monroe's death in a televised press conference.[20] "Now that the final toxicological report and that of the psychiatric consultants have been received and considered," he told the listening audience, "it is my conclusion that the death of Marilyn Monroe was caused by a self-administered overdose of sedative drugs and that the mode of death is a probable suicide."[20] No one thought his announcement would be the final word on the matter, as numerous conspiracy theories immediately began to emerge.

While I agree with Curphey's conclusion that Monroe had intentionally swallowed a large number of two different types of sedative drugs, I wouldn't have qualified her suicide as "probable" since it left room for doubt. Some people expressed their frustration, thinking if help had arrived in time, Monroe could have been rescued from her suicide attempt, as had been done in the past. Others speculated that Monroe's death was an unfortunate accident. They suggested Monroe must have lost count of how many pills she ingested, or her physicians didn't coordinate their prescriptions, with one giving her an enema of chloral hydrate when the other had already given her oral doses of pentobarbital.[21] None of these theories was true. Nevertheless, Monroe's friends continued to believe her death was an accident, pointing to evidence her career was on an upswing. It was just wishful thinking.[22]

Life and Career

To better understand what led Monroe to commit suicide, one must first understand her life. Who was Norma Jeane Mortenson, the woman who became known as Marilyn Monroe?

When Monroe was born, her mother, Gladys, named her Norma Jeane after Norma Talmadge, a popular screen idol of the 1920s, but her grandmother christened her Norma Jeane Baker.[23] It was only later that Ben Lyon, a casting director at Twentieth Century-Fox, suggested she change her name to Marilyn, and she selected Monroe, her mother's maiden name, for her surname.[24] On her birth certificate, Monroe's father is identified as Martin Edward Mortenson, Gladys's second husband, but most biographers now believe her father was actually C. Stanley Gifford, one of her mother's coworkers at Consolidated Film Industries.[25]

Monroe's mother and maternal grandparents were all in mental institutions, and her uncle on her mother's side was diagnosed with paranoid schizophrenia, so Monroe was always worried she had inherited a genetic predisposition for mental illness.[26] It was because of her mental illness that Gladys placed her daughter in foster care when she was only twelve days old.[27] But when Monroe was seven, she moved back home, only to be placed in a foster home for a second time when her mother was again institutionalized—only this time, it was for the rest of her life.[27] Later, Monroe would be placed in an orphanage and then with family friends until she reached her sixteenth birthday, when she married a neighbor's son.[27]

It was while Monroe worked for an aviation defense contractor, after her husband had joined the Merchant Marines, that David Conover, a photographer with the United States Army Air Forces' First Motion Picture Unit, who was on assignment for the military magazine *Yank*, saw the young, charismatic, and very photogenic eighteen-year-old and decided to feature her in his article to boost the morale of soldiers overseas.[28] "Her eyes held something that touched and intrigued me," he said when asked why he selected Monroe for the magazine article.[29] From that moment on, Monroe's photos began to appear regularly in *Yank* and *Stars and Stripes*.[29] By 1946, her image was in most of the popular pin-up photo magazines.[29]

After she received a modeling assignment for *Rayve* shampoo, Monroe straightened her natural brunette curls and lightened her hair to a reddish-blonde, eventually lightening it to a golden honey-blonde color.[29] Later, when she was at Columbia Pictures, she colored her hair further to what became her signature platinum-blonde.[29]

When Lyon was introduced to Monroe, he immediately recognized that although she didn't have any experience in front of the camera, her charisma and charm would be magnified on the big screen.[29] He arranged for a screen test, and a week later, Darryl Zanuck, the head of production at Twentieth Century-Fox, signed Monroe to a six-month contract.[29] It was soon followed by a movie deal.[29]

Monroe was anxious to make it as a serious, dramatic actress, but her physical attributes—exceptional good looks and hourglass figure—and her pin-up photos always overshadowed her dream. Twentieth Century-Fox was reluctant to cast Monroe in dramatic roles, fearful the public wouldn't accept her in anything less than as a "blonde bombshell" in comedies.[30] However, in 1950, Monroe got her big break when she secured a coveted role in the John Huston film *The Asphalt Jungle* and followed it with a performance in *All About Eve*.[30] Then, in 1952, she was selected to play a cunning adulteress who plots to murder her neurotic husband in the film *Niagara*.[31] Reviews of Monroe's acting were complimentary, but she gained a reputation for being difficult on the set.[31]

When Johnny Hyde, Monroe's agent at the William Morris Agency, suddenly died, Monroe became so despondent that several days after his funeral, she was discovered unconscious after swallowing a bottle of sleeping pills.[31] It would be her first of several attempts at suicide.

By now, Monroe's popularity was at an all-time high, mostly for her pin-up photos and her *Golden Dream* calendar, in which she posed nude.[31] Her unbridled audacity was reminiscent of Mae West, an actress of the 1930s who was famous for her sassiness. Once, when reporters asked Monroe what she wore to bed, she deadpanned, "Chanel No. 5."[31] The public loved it!

In *The Seven Year Itch,* the scene that made an indelible impression was of Monroe standing over a New York City subway grating and saying to her costar after they exited the Trans-Lux Fifty-Second Street Theatre, where they saw the horror film *The Creature from the Black Lagoon*, "Ooh, do you feel the breeze from the subway? Isn't it delicious?"—as the wind from a train passing beneath the grating blew her skirt above her hips, exposing her long, slender legs and momentarily titillating the audience, before she held her dress down, preventing it from rising any further.[32] The photo of Monroe standing on the subway grating became one of the most iconic Hollywood photos of all time, and the film, which was the perfect vehicle to show off Monroe's talent and personality and to instill her innocence and sexuality into a character, became one of the biggest box office successes that year. [32] As for the dress Monroe wore in that famous scene, it sold at auction in 2011 for $4.6 million.[33]

Monroe received some of her best reviews for her performance in *Bus Stop*.[34] And her next film, *Some Like It Hot*, quickly became a classic for which she won a Golden Globe Award for best actress in a comedy or musical.[35] Later, in *The Misfits*, she played a recently divorced woman opposite Clark Gable, an accomplished actor who made his mark in *Gone with the Wind*, a film set during the Civil War.[35]

Something's Got to Give was Monroe's last but never finished film.[36] She often appeared hours late on the set, claiming she was too sick to perform.[37] But despite her supposed illness, Monroe appeared in a white fur coat at Madison Square Garden in New York City to seductively sing "Happy Birthday, Mr. President" in a sultry and intimate voice at the forty-fifth birthday party for John F. Kennedy, president of the United States.[38] People would later remember Monroe for the sheer, flesh-colored, skintight dress she wore the night she sang for the president. It sparkled because of the twenty-five hundred rhinestones sewn into the fabric.[39] It was said Monroe didn't wear anything underneath the dress and it was stitched together only after she put it on.[40] The dress sold at auction in 2016 for $4.8 million, topping the one Monroe wore in *The Seven Year Itch*.[41] For the studio, it was just too much to accept, and on June 8, 1962, Monroe was fired from the film.[42] Three months later, she was dead.

Conclusion

Like most suicides, Monroe's death cannot be explained by a single line on a death certificate. Psychologists would surely agree that if Monroe's death was a suicide, then many years of living in foster care and an orphanage had undoubtedly contributed to her unhappiness and untimely death.

That Monroe never knew who her father was may have been the reason why she had gravitated toward much older men. Both Joe DiMaggio, a conservative, low-key baseball hero, and Miller, the well-respected playwright, were eleven to twelve years her senior when she married them.[43] In addition, Hyde, Monroe's manager to whom she was very close, as well as Gable, an actor whom she idolized, were thirty-one years and twenty-five years older than she was, respectively.[43] That she loved children but could never have any of her own surely must have further contributed to Monroe's mounting sorrow.[43]

I would rather remember Monroe for her life than her death. Besides entertaining and giving of herself to the public through her talent as an actress and singer and her pin-up photos, Monroe was a strong supporter of the military.[44] On one occasion, she interrupted her honeymoon to entertain the troops in South Korea, despite freezing temperatures that most likely contributed to her developing pneumonia.[45] "It was the best thing that ever happened to me," she later said.[46] And when the owner of the popular Mocambo nightclub in West Hollywood refused to feature Ella Fitzgerald, the greatest jazz singer of all time, because she was African American, Monroe offered to sit at the front table every night if he would book Fitzgerald, which he promptly did.[47] "She was ahead of her time," Fitzgerald said.[47]

In an age when the film industry was controlled by the male-dominated studio system, Monroe was one of its early unrecognized feminists. Dissatisfied with the parts she was given at Twentieth Century-Fox, she formed her own Marilyn Monroe Production Company. Within a year, Twentieth Century-Fox realized their loss and begged Monroe to return to its fold, agreeing to all of her demands—creative control that included approval of the story, director, and cinematographer and an increase in salary to $100,000 per film, permission to make films with independent producers and other studios, and to be cast only in top-notch, "A-films."[48] It was an unprecedented outcome that opened the way for other established actors to seek the same level of control over their careers. The *Los Angeles Mirror News* reported it was "One of the greatest single triumphs ever won by an actress."[49] *Look* magazine described the win as "an example of the individual against the herd for years to come."[49] Overnight, Monroe was no longer seen as a dumb blonde but as a shrewd businesswoman.

Much has been said about Monroe, but of one thing I think we can all agree. There has never been anyone like her. In life, Monroe was an icon, but in death, she became a legend. The only thing she ever wanted was to be respected by her peers as a serious dramatic actress. She had won a Golden Globe Award as well as Italy's prestigious David di Donatello Prize and France's Crystal Star Award.[50] But the one award that would have solidified her worth to and admiration by the industry to which she devoted her adult life, an Oscar, had eluded her forever.[50] And while millions of photos of Monroe were sold worldwide, and her thirty films grossed more than $200 million, the studios eventually turned their collective backs on her. Monroe's unbelievable beauty and vulnerability, qualities that endeared her to her fans, were the very reason why the studios couldn't accept her as a serious dramatic actress, a status she so eagerly wanted but would never achieve. Nevertheless, in spite of her well-publicized feuds with directors and studios, the public loved and admired Monroe for her talent, sex appeal, singing voice, and special walk, but it wasn't enough.

Through the years, many women have tried to imitate Monroe, including Mamie Van Doren, Jayne Mansfield, Anna Nicole Smith, Lady Gaga, and Gwen Stefani. [51] Elton John penned *Candle in the Wind* as a tribute to Monroe, and The Beatles prominently displayed

Monroe's likeness on the sleeve of their album *Sgt. Pepper's Lonely Hearts Club Band.*[52]

Monroe was more than just a beautiful, platinum-haired woman with a curvaceous, hourglass figure. She was a sex symbol, some even called her a blonde bombshell, but she was more than a goddess to be put on a pedestal. With her breathy voice and ready smile, Monroe seemed childlike and approachable, exuding charm and understanding, yet vulnerable to the core. And when she married DiMaggio and Miller, neither one of whom was extraordinarily handsome, Monroe cemented the notion that no woman was beyond the reach of the average looking man. But in the end, the very attributes that made Monroe famous were what brought about her early demise.

CHAPTER 3

Jimi Hendrix

Died September 18, 1970

JIMI HENDRIX, ONE of the best guitar-playing musicians of his time, attended a party in London on Thursday evening, September 17, 1970, where he took at least one amphetamine pill.[1] Later that night, Hendrix went to the apartment of Monika Dannemann, a German figure skater whom he had befriended nine months earlier, when he was performing at a concert in Dusseldorf, Germany.[1] When he arrived at the Samarkand Hotel on Landsdown Crescent where Dannemann was staying, she cooked him a meal, after which they drank a bottle of wine together and spent the evening talking and listening to music.[2] However, at about 1:45 a.m., Hendrix wanted to "see some people," so Dannemann drove him to his meeting place and picked him up again at about three o'clock.[2] Upon their return, she made Hendrix a tuna fish sandwich, but he only took a couple of bites before they went to bed.[3]

At approximately seven o'clock on Friday morning, Dannemann took a sleeping pill, only to awake about three and a half hours later.[3] "I wanted some cigarettes," she said at Hendrix's inquest. She looked to see if Hendrix was awake, but he was still asleep.[4] Determined to go out, Dannemann looked at Hendrix again and saw "there was sick [vomit] on his nose and mouth," as she told the coroner.[4] "I tried to wake him up but couldn't."[4]

After first calling a friend for advice, Dannemann summoned an ambulance.[4] It arrived within twenty minutes. Hendrix was transported to St. Mary Abbots Hospital in the Kensington section of London, but tragically, he died along the way.[5] He was twenty-seven years old.[5]

The Autopsy

Police did not suspect foul play in Hendrix's death.[6] While the autopsy and toxicology reports were not available for review, articles published at the time noted that Hendrix's autopsy was conducted by Professor Donald Teare three days after Hendrix died.[7]

Teare had a well-respected reputation as an accomplished forensic pathologist. In 1958, he was the first to publish a description of hypertrophic cardiomyopathy, a condition in which a portion of the heart becomes thickened so the heart doesn't pump blood efficiently, a leading cause of sudden death in young athletes.[8] Along with Keith Simpson and Francis Camps, the three pathologists conducted the autopsies on almost all of the suspicious deaths in London and its environs.[8]

At the inquest, Teare reported he found no evidence that Hendrix was an intravenous drug abuser.[9] "The normal signs are marks on hands and arms [but] in this case, there were no marks whatsoever," Teare said.[9] However, he didn't exclude the possibility Hendrix had been taking cocaine by nasal insufflation or was addicted to pharmaceuticals taken orally. By his own admission, Hendrix had tried "just about everything."[10]

According to Dannemann, Hendrix had swallowed nine of her Vesparax sleeping pills, a combination of two barbiturates, secobarbital and brallobarbital, and the antihistamine, hydroxyzine.[11] "They are in packets of ten and I thought he had taken the lot, but a policeman found one on the floor," she testified.[11] "The question why Hendrix took so many sleeping tablets cannot be safely answered," said Gavin Thurston, the coroner of West London.[11]

Cause and Manner of Death

Thurston concluded that the cause of Hendrix's death was inhalation of vomit due to barbiturate intoxication after having taken a barbiturate overdose.[12] This is consistent with the well-recognized potential harmful complications of aspiration of food, drink, or stomach contents. Sometimes the damage to the lungs could be severe. At other times, aspiration can increase the risk of pneumonia. In rare cases, especially when the nervous system is depressed by drugs, as was the case with Hendrix, aspiration of vomit can cause death.

The manner of Hendrix's death was "an open verdict," a term used in the United Kingdom, equivalent to "undetermined" in the United States.[13] It was based on insufficient evidence to prove Hendrix had committed suicide, presumably because of the absence of a suicide note and a lack of evidence his death was an accident. [13] However, while there are many examples of deaths caused by a drug overdose that were determined to be an accident, when suicide was a possibility, despite the absence of a suicide note, as with Marilyn Monroe and Anna Nicole Smith, a psychological autopsy was conducted to establish intent. In Monroe's case, her death was ruled a suicide, whereas Smith's death was an accident. However, in Hendrix's case, a psychological autopsy apparently was never performed. Also, there was no evidence Hendrix showed suicidal tendencies in the days leading up to his death. In my opinion, since the immediate cause of Hendrix's death was inhalation of vomit, the manner of his death should have been labeled an accident with barbiturate intoxication as a contributing factor.

Nearly fifty years after Hendrix died, a popular twenty-seven-year-old professional baseball player for the Los Angeles Angels, Tyler Skaggs, also died from aspiration of gastric contents caused by drug intoxication. [14] However, unlike with Hendrix, the manner of Skaggs's death was ruled an accident.[14]

In December 1993, Kathy Etchingham, Hendrix's former girlfriend, asked British Attorney General Nicholas Lyell to reopen the investigation into Hendrix's death.[15] "He was in the wrong place at the wrong time and with the wrong people," she was quoted as saying.[16] But three months after she submitted her request, Lyell rejected Etchingham's demand, noting there simply wasn't sufficient new evidence to warrant a new inquest.[17]

Life and Career

Born in Seattle, Washington, in 1942 to a seventeen-year-old mother, Hendrix's early years were difficult.[18] Part black, part Cherokee Indian, and part Mexican, Hendrix was sent to live with relatives in Berkeley, California, while his father was off fighting in World War II and his mother battled alcoholism.[19] When the war ended, his parents divorced, and Hendrix went to live with his father.[20]

Hendrix received his first acoustic guitar when he was in his midteens.[21] Being left-handed, he taught himself to strum with both hands and joined a band, the Velvetones.[22] The following year, his father bought him his first electric guitar, at which time Hendrix joined another band, the Rocking Kings.[23]

In the middle of his senior year, Hendrix dropped out of Garfield High School and enlisted in the United States Army.[23] Ten years later, the school awarded him an honorary diploma.[24]

After his military service ended, Hendrix became a session musician, backing performers such as Little Richard, B.B. King, and Sam Cooke.[25] When he tired of playing backup for other musicians, he formed his own band, Jimmy James and the Blue Flames.[26] The band played at various clubs on MacDougal Street in

New York City's Greenwich Village.[27] It was there that Hendrix was introduced to marijuana, amphetamine, and cocaine.[28]

One day in the mid-1960s, when Jimmy James and the Blue Flames band were performing at the Café Wha?, a favorite Greenwich Village spot for upcoming musicians such as Bob Dylan, Bruce Springsteen, and Peter, Paul, and Mary, John Hammond Jr., a singer and guitar player who was appearing at Café Au Go Go, a nearby popular venue, asked Hendrix to play backup for him, to which Hendrix promptly agreed.[29] At the end of the show, Hammond invited Hendrix to play Bo Didley's "I'm the Man."[30] Linda Keith, girlfriend of Keith Richards of the Rolling Stones, was there that night. She was so impressed with Hendrix that she mentioned him to Chas Chandler, an English musician, record producer, and manager.[30] Chandler agreed to manage Hendrix and invited him to England, where he formed his new band, Jimi Hendrix Experience.[31] The band released its first single, "Hey Joe," in England in October 1966. It was a huge hit, peaking at number six on the British music charts.[31] Other successful singles soon followed, including "Purple Haze" and "The Wind Cries Mary."[32]

In the summer of 1967, Hendrix delighted people attending the Monterey International Pop Festival with his innovative musical style and his playing of "Wild

Thing" with his teeth, culminating his performance by lighting his guitar on fire.[33] Pete Johnson of Warner Brothers, speaking about the Jimi Hendrix Experience, proclaimed, "Their appearance at the Festival was magical. The way they looked, the way they performed and the way they sounded were light years away from anything anyone had seen before."[34]

Two years later, Hendrix was arrested for possession of heroin and hashish while crossing the Canadian border.[34] At his trial, he claimed a fan had given him the bag and he didn't look inside or know what was in it.[34] He admitted, however, he had tried "just about everything" in the past, from marijuana to cocaine, but had never taken heroin.[35] After deliberating for three days, the jury found Hendrix innocent of all charges.[36]

Three months after his trial, Hendrix's performance was the final act on the morning of the fourth and final day of Woodstock.[37] By the time he took the stage, there were only 25,000 of the original 400,000 spectators remaining to see the closing number.[37] No one was disappointed. Hendrix's searing rendition of "The Star-Spangled Banner," the national anthem of the United States, was not only mesmerizing, it demonstrated his unique talent as a musician and performer.[38] When he reached the line, "And the rocket's red glare, the bombs bursting in air," Hendrix ramped up his amplifiers. The music produced by his guitar mimicked the sound of bombs being dropped from B-52 bombers and exploding over Vietnam. It was as moving and as powerful an antiwar expression by an artist as the 1937 painting, *Guernica*, by Pablo Picasso, the famous Spanish painter.

Conclusion

Recognized by his peers as a musical genius, Hendrix was considered by many to be the greatest guitar player of all time. "Absolutely the best guitar player that ever lived," said Neil Young, an American singer-songwriter and a former collaborator with Crosby, Stills & Nash.[39] "He played just about every style you could think of, and not in a flashy way," said Eric Clapton, an English rock and blues guitarist, singer, and songwriter and a former member of The Yardbirds and Cream.[40] But despite his virtuosity, fame, and undeniable success, Hendrix only had one top-forty hit in the United States.[41]

"Music is so important," Hendrix said.[42] "Music doesn't lie. Music is going to change the world."[42] He felt that while drugs can open up a person's mind, "music can [also] do that, you know, and you don't need any drugs."[42] Ironically, Hendrix died from complications caused by a drug overdose.

"The moment I feel that I don't have anything more to give musically," Hendrix once said, "that's when I won't be found on this planet ... because if I don't have anything to communicate through my music, then there is nothing for me to live for."[43] No one would dispute Hendrix had much more to give. "The story of life is quicker than the wink of an eye," he proclaimed.[44] "The story of love is hello and goodbye. Until we meet again."[44]

The world mourned when Hendrix, a shy, personable, and charming man with a good sense of humor who could play the guitar left-handed, right-handed, upside down, and even with his teeth joined the Twenty-Seven Club, a group of prominent musicians who died at the age of twenty-seven, whose members include Janis Joplin, Jim Morrison of the Doors, Amy Winehouse, Brian Jones of the Rolling Stones, and Kurt Cobain of Nirvana.[45] However, Hendrix would have undoubtedly implored his fans not to be sad. "Sadness is for when a baby is born into this heavy world," he claimed.[46] "Once you are dead, you are made for life."[47]

CHAPTER 4

Janis Joplin

Died October 4, 1970

JANIS JOPLIN, THE twenty-seven-year-old singer with the blues-inspired vocals, had booked a room at the Landmark Motor Hotel on Franklin Avenue in Hollywood, a boutique hotel conveniently located on Sunset Boulevard and where many famous celebrities, including members of the Rat Pack and the Jefferson Airplane, had previously stayed.[1] At 6:00 p.m. on Sunday, October 4, 1970, she failed to show up at Sunset Sound Studios to complete recording what would turn out to be her biggest-selling album, *Pearl*.[2] It included the song "Me & Bobby McGee," originally sung by Roger

Miller and cowritten by American singer-songwriter Kris Kristofferson and songwriter Fred Foster.[2] Since Joplin wasn't answering her phone, John Cooke, a road manager for the Full Tilt Boogie Band, Joplin's third and newest band, went to fetch her.

Cook arrived at the Landmark at about seven o'clock. He was suspicious when he saw the drapes to Joplin's first-floor hotel room fully drawn. In addition, Joplin's customized 1964 Porsche 356 Cabriolet, painted in psychedelic colors, was parked in the outdoor parking lot instead of in its usual spot in the garage, which Cook thought was odd.[3] The car, which Joplin bought in 1968 for $3,500, would be sold at auction five years later for $1.76 million.[4] Knocking loudly on Joplin's door, Cook called out her name, but she didn't respond.[5] With the help of the hotel's manager, he entered the room only to find Joplin lying on the floor between the bed and the nightstand, her lips bloody and her nose broken, with four one-dollar bills and two quarters clutched tightly in her hand.[5] On the side table was a pack of Marlboro cigarettes.[5] It was obvious, Cooke would write in his memoir, "she got change for a five, bought cigarettes for fifty cents from the machine in the lobby, came back to the room, sat down, and keeled over before she could light one."[6]

When police arrived, they discovered Joplin deceased with several fresh needle marks on her left arm.[7] They determined she had been dead for approximately twelve hours.[7] In one of the hotel's dresser drawers, police found a spoon and a hypodermic needle. In a wastepaper basket, they found a red balloon containing a white powder.[7]

The Autopsy

A deputy medical examiner of the county of Los Angeles, Dr. David M. Katsuyama was a board-certified clinical and anatomical pathologist with more than ten years' experience.[8] He had performed more than five hundred autopsies by the time he was selected to conduct Joplin's autopsy.[8]

Katsuyama had just finished performing the autopsies on several of Charles Manson's victims, the self-proclaimed leader of a hippie "family," and his three followers.[9] The gruesome killings of Sharon Tate, an actress who was eight and a half months pregnant, at her rented home, along with four other people, as well as of Leno and Rosemary LaBianca, who were killed the following day, had captivated the public's imagination for days.[10] Now, based on the circumstances surrounding Joplin's final hours, Katsuyama suspected her death was probably caused by a drug overdose. My plan was to

review the autopsy findings and to critically evaluate
Katsuyama's conclusions.

There was no evidence that violence or trauma had
contributed to Joplin's death.[11] Her bloodied lips and
broken nose most likely occurred when she fell in her
hotel room. Nevertheless, the tattoo of a bracelet around
her left wrist, another of a flower behind her right heel,
and a third of a heart next to her left breast were in sharp
contrast with the self-inflicted numerous needle marks
on both of Joplin's arms.[11] In addition, the fresh needle
marks on her left arm and the small amount of foamy
material in the upper portion of her trachea were a clear
indication Joplin had probably died from an overdose of
an opioid drug.[11]

On internal examination, Joplin's cardiovascular
system appeared within normal limits. The heart was
of the expected size and weight for a female of Joplin's
age, and the aorta, as well as its branching arteries, had
a minimal amount of plaque, not enough to significantly
impede blood flow or to have caused a heart attack.
[11] And while there was some evidence of congestion
and pulmonary edema, or fluid in the lungs, it was not
an unusual finding, especially when heroin use was
suspected.[11]

What I found fascinating in the autopsy report was
the description of Joplin's liver as "yellowish-brown with

a glistening surface" that Katsuyama labeled as fatty metamorphosis.[12] While this condition is commonly found in people with a history of severe alcoholism, as was seen in Errol Flynn, it can also occur in people who suffered from morbid obesity or type 2 diabetes. However, Joplin wasn't overweight, and she wasn't a diabetic. And yet, although she was very young and normally wouldn't have been expected to have had a fatty liver, the finding was consistent with her long history of alcohol abuse, sometimes swigging whiskey straight out of the bottle, as she did during her performance at Woodstock when she was noticeably inebriated.[13]

Cause and Manner of Death

Police determined that Joplin bought heroin shortly before she died. However, what she apparently didn't realize at the time was that the drug was much more potent than any heroin she had obtained in the past.[14] It wasn't surprising, therefore, that toxicology analysis identified morphine, a pharmacologically active metabolite of heroin, in Joplin's blood.[15] However, what was especially disturbing was how large the amount of morphine was, substantial enough to have been within the range previously reported in people who had died from a heroin overdose.[15] Invariably, after the heroin

49

entered Joplin's bloodstream, it was rapidly metabolized to morphine. The morphine, in turn, bound to areas of the brain responsible for respiration, with death following from respiratory depression. It was a painless way to die but one that could have probably been prevented had Joplin been treated with naloxone, a recognized antidote for an opioid overdose.

Joplin's blood also contained alcohol, the concentration of which was 38 percent above the current legal limit for drivers in the United States.[16] At this level, it would have enhanced the central nervous system depressant and sedative effects of heroin and morphine.

Dr. Noguchi had replaced Curphey in 1967 as the chief medical examiner-coroner of the county of Los Angeles. Now, based on the autopsy findings and results of toxicology tests, he declared that Joplin died from acute heroin-morphine intoxication brought about by an injection of a heroin overdose, and the manner of her death was an accident.[16] I found no reason to disagree with his conclusions.

Life and Career

As a teenager, Joplin was an overweight, acne-skinned "ugly duckling" who dressed like a beatnik, was bullied in high school, and listened to music by Bessie Smith and Leadbelly, among others.[17] "They laughed me out of class, out of town, and out of state," Joplin told Dick Cavett about her high school experience, in the second of her three television interviews shortly before her death.[18]

Although she attended Lamar State College of Technology and the University of Texas at Austin, Joplin never finished college, opting instead to sing the blues at local Texas bars and in San Francisco coffeehouses where, coincidentally, she began to abuse amphetamine, an upper, and alcohol, a downer, especially Southern Comfort whiskey.[19]

In 1966, Joplin teamed up with the high-energy Haight-Ashbury band Big Brother and the Holding Company and soon became its lead singer.[19] "All of a sudden, someone threw me in front of this rock and roll band and I decided then and there that was it," Joplin said at the time.[20] "I never wanted to do anything else." A year later, she appeared at the Monterey Pop Festival where her raspy singing of the rhythm and blues song "Ball & Chain" was well received.[21] By the time she performed at Woodstock in 1969, Joplin was addicted to heroin and alcohol, two drugs that depress the central nervous system, thereby ensuring that her reputation as the "Queen of Psychedelic Soul" was well on its way.[22]

Conclusion

According to Jack Doyle of *The Pop History Dig*, a magazine-styled website about contemporary culture and popular history, Joplin was a "shooting star who burned white hot for five short years."[23] When he heard of Joplin's passing, Clive Davis, president of Columbia Records, said "She, more than anyone else at Monterey, made me intensely aware and excited about the new and future direction of music."[24]

Heroin cut Joplin's life short before she achieved her full potential. Weeks earlier, Jimi Hendrix, another rock and roll musical genius, also died from a drug overdose. According to the National Institute on Drug Abuse, or NIDA, people who use heroin report feeling a "rush," a surge of euphoria. However, when the drug is taken in an overdose, it can cause breathing to slow down or even to stop, which could then lead to hypoxia, a condition in which the amount of oxygen reaching the brain is drastically reduced.[25] This can cause permanent brain damage, coma, and even death from respiratory depression.[25]

In death, Joplin joined a long list of celebrities who died from a heroin overdose. Among them were Dee Dee Ramone of the Ramones and Sid Vicious of the Sex Pistols. Jim Morrison of the Doors died of a heart attack, but his cardiac event was determined to be due to his chronic use of heroin. Nevertheless, while Joplin used illicit drugs and died because of them, it should not overshadow her musical legacy or define who she was.

CHAPTER 5

Cass Elliot

Died July 29, 1974

CASS ELLIOT COMPLETED a two-week singing engagement at the London Paladium on July 27, 1974, a venue often compared to New York City's Carnegie Hall. [1] Since 1968, the year the Mamas and the Papas broke up, she had been trying to emerge as a well-respected and talented solo artist. On her last night at the Paladium, Elliot was elated the audience had given her a standing ovation. "[Cass] felt she had finally made the transition from Mama Cass," said Michelle Philips, a former band member of the Mamas and the Papas. [1]

The following evening, Elliot attended a cocktail party at the home of Mick Jagger of the Rolling Stones. Her friends and staff visited her apartment in the Mayfair section of London on July 29, but they didn't enter her room, assuming she was asleep. Unable to make contact, Elliot's secretary went to her apartment nd found Elliot dead.[2] She was thirty-three years old.

The Autopsy

Professor Keith Simpson, one of the most renowned forensic pathologists in England, performed Elliot's autopsy.[3] Elliot's death certificate noted she died from "fatty myocardial degeneration due to obesity."[4] According to one report, a third of her heart muscle had degenerated.[5] "Cassie literally died of a broken heart," Denny Doherty said when he heard of Elliot's death.[5]

Cause and Manner of Death

Police found a half-eaten sandwich on Elliot's nightstand, which quickly led a rumor to circulate that Elliot died by choking on a sandwich. However, it wasn't true. The autopsy showed clear airways with no evidence of food in Elliot's throat or trachea.[6] Also, no drugs were detected in her system.[7]

Elliot had been battling her weight ever since she was seven years old.[7] Bobby Roberts, her former manager, claimed, "She was overweight, but she carried it off like she was a beauty queen."[7] According to John Phillip, Elliot tried to lose weight with various diets on several occasions.[8]

Based on a review of the available records, Simpson concluded, and I agreed, that the cause of Elliot's death was congestive heart failure due to obesity. The manner of death was natural.

Life and Career

Elliot spent her early years in Baltimore, Maryland.[9] In her senior year in high school, she performed in a touring production of *The Music Man*, as well as off Broadway. By the early 1960s, she formed a folk trio known as the Big 3.[10] The group recorded two albums and appeared on *The Tonight Show with Johnny Carson, Hootenanny,* and *The Danny Kay Show.*[11] However, by 1964, the trio disbanded.[12]

After the Big 3, Elliot formed a new group called the Mugwumps composed of four singers, one of whom was Doherty.[12] When the Mugwumps split up, Doherty joined two other singers, John and Michelle Phillips, in the Journeymen. They considered inviting Elliot to become a member of the group, but John Phillips was opposed to the idea, afraid that Elliot's weight, by some estimates reaching up to three hundred pounds, would create an image problem for the group.[13] However, when he heard Elliot sing, he became convinced she would not only be a great asset because of her contralto voice but would serve as a contrast for the delicate and beautiful blonde soprano, Michelle Phillips.[14]

In the mid-1960s, Elliot joined Doherty and the Phillips, and they renamed their group the Mamas and the Papas.[15] According to Doherty, the group's name was inspired by members of the motorcycle club, Hells Angels, who said on *The Tonight Show* that they called their women "mamas."[16] With its unduplicated harmonious sound, the Mamas and the Papas sang together for only three years (1965–1968), but during that time, the group had a series of top-ten hits, all written by John Phillips, including "Monday, Monday," "California Dreamin'," "I Saw Her Again," and "Dedicated to the One I Love." [17] Elliot's powerful and distinctive voice can clearly be heard above the others as she, along with Doherty's tenor voice, often carried the tune.[18]

Elliot's solo career began in 1968 with what became her signature theme song, "Dream a Little Dream of Me."[19] Sometime around October of that year, she went on a six-month crash diet and lost one hundred pounds before she made her solo debut at Caesar's Palace in Las Vegas.[20] However, shortly thereafter, she regained fifty of those pounds and developed a stomach ulcer and throat problems.[20] "I would say the world's in terrible shape," Elliot once joked, "but I'm afraid the world would say, 'Look who's talking.'"[21]

Within six short years, Elliot had several hits, including "It's Getting Better," "Make Your Own Kind of Music," and "New World Coming." However, none of the songs was as popular as the ones she sang with the Mamas and the Papas.[22] She also appeared on several television variety shows, guest-hosted *The Tonight Show*, and had successful performances in Las Vegas.[23] Trying to shed her "Mama Cass" persona, her final album, released in 1973, was entitled *Don't Call Me Mama Anymore*.[24] "I never created the Big Mama image," Elliot said in her final interview.[25] "The public does it for you."

In 1998, fourteen years after she died, Elliot was inducted into the Rock and Roll Hall of Fame, along with the three other members of the Mamas and the Papas—Doherty and John and Michelle Phillips.[26] She "opened the door for others like Janis Joplin and Grace Slick of Jefferson Airplane," Annie Nightingale, Britain's first female DJ on Radio 1, said of Elliot.[27]

Conclusion

Obesity is a recognized risk factor for congestive heart failure, a leading cause of morbidity and mortality. When congestive heart failure is caused entirely or predominantly by obesity, it is known as "obesity cardiomyopathy," previously called "fatty myocardial degeneration due to obesity."[28] Studies have shown an association between obesity and ventricular heart chamber dysfunction, an increase in blood pressure or hypertension, as well as coronary artery disease, structural and functional changes in the heart, various metabolic changes, and heart failure.[28] People with obesity cardiomyopathy die mainly due to sudden death caused by progressive congestive heart failure.[29]

"Being fat sets you apart," Elliot once said to William Otterburn-Hall of *Rolling Stone* magazine, "but luckily I was bright with it; I had an IQ of 165 … I got into the habit of being independent, and the habit became a design for living."[30]

CHAPTER 6

Elvis Presley

Died August 16, 1977

ON AUGUST 16, 1977, Elvis Presley, known as the "King of Rock and Roll," told Ginger, his new live-in girlfriend, that he would be reading in the master bathroom of his Graceland mansion. "Don't fall asleep" in there, she told him.[1] However, when he didn't come out, she became concerned and opened the bathroom door, only to find Presley lying on the floor with his eyes fixed, staring straight ahead.[2] Presley was rushed to Baptist Memorial Hospital and was pronounced dead at 3:30 p.m. He was forty-two years old.

The Autopsy

Presley's autopsy took two hours and was conducted in the late afternoon, the same day he died.[2] A team of nine pathologists from the Baptist Memorial Hospital performed the autopsy.[3] Foul play was not suspected, nor was there evidence Presley had suffered a stroke or a concussion.[4]

An internal examination revealed that Presley's cardiovascular system was significantly compromised. His heart was enlarged, weighing about twice as much as a normal heart, mainly because of an enlarged left ventricle heart chamber.[5] In addition, the coronary arteries and aorta had significant accumulation of atherosclerotic plaque.[5] Other autopsy findings included evidence of chronic constipation, undoubtedly due to Presley's excessive use of opioids, as well as an enlarged colon, diabetes, glaucoma, and a mildly enlarged, congested spleen.[6] As for the enlarged liver, it was due to fatty metamorphosis, a condition often found in alcoholics. However, unlike Errol Flynn and Janis Joplin, who drank liquor to excess over many years and also suffered from a fatty liver, Presley did not drink alcohol. Most likely, his fatty metamorphosis was due to his extreme obesity.[7]

Dr. Jerry Francisco, the medical examiner of Shelby County in Memphis, Tennessee, completed the autopsy at about eight o'clock in the evening. Presley died from a cardiac arrhythmia, and drugs did not play a role in his death, said Francisco.[8] His announcement may have been premature, however, especially since an arrhythmia cannot be diagnosed after death and toxicology tests had not yet been performed.

Cause and Manner of Death

Presley's blood was analyzed for the presence of drugs at the Center for Human Toxicology at the University of Utah. The tests identified eight different pharmaceuticals, all with sedative properties, including codeine, an opioid drug, four tranquilizers—methaqualone, diazepam, ethchlorvynol, and ethinamate—as well as three barbiturates—pentobarbital, phenobarbital, and butabarbital.[9] "All the drugs were in a range consistent with therapy and therapeutic requirements for known conditions of illnesses," Dr. Bryan S. Finkle, director of the Center for Human Toxicology told reporters.[10] "Had these drugs not been present, he still would have died," Francisco chimed in.[11]

Without the ability to review the toxicology report, it was impossible to determine whether any of the drugs found in Presley's system were in the overdose range. However, the presence of eight different central nervous system depressant drugs in Presley's blood, a prime example of polypharmacy, undoubtedly was a contributing factor in his death.

Sometime after Presley died, the investigative report of his death was made public. "Presley died from hypertensive cardiovascular disease with arteriosclerotic heart disease as a contributing factor," Francisco concluded.[12] The manner of death was natural.[12] In other words, according to Francisco, Presley died from a heart attack.

The final autopsy report was not issued until months after the autopsy was completed. However, the document was sealed for fifty years.[12] By not sharing the coroner's final conclusions, it led to much speculation, with many people believing Presley died from a drug overdose. Fans organized "Presley is alive" movements, and various Presley impersonators began to flood Las Vegas and Memphis.

In 1994, partly due to public pressure, the state of Tennessee retained Dr. Joseph Davis to reexamine Presley's autopsy findings. "There is nothing in any of the data that supports a death from drugs," Davis declared. [13] "In fact, everything points to a sudden, violent heart attack. It takes hours to die from drugs, [but] based on the position of the body, Presley must have died by the time he hit the floor. In addition, he was significantly overweight, which put a significant strain on his heart, and there was no pulmonary edema, fluid in the lungs, a sign of a drug overdose."[14]

In his report, Davis noted that Presley died with his pajama bottoms pulled all the way down.[15] In addition, Ginger, Presley's girlfriend, said that when she found Presley in the bathroom, he looked as if his entire body had completely frozen in a seated position and that he had fallen forward from the commode.[16] Based on these descriptions, as well as published reports of the autopsy findings, I concluded that Presley most likely suffered a heart-related event, probably an arrhythmia, an opinion shared by Francisco and Dr. Forest Tennant, an expert later retained by Dr. George Nichopoulos, Presley's personal physician, for his subsequent trial.[17]

Presley was already at a significant risk for sudden death from an arrhythmia due to his enlarged heart. When he strained on the commode due to his severe constipation, he undoubtedly put great pressure on his heart and aorta and most likely triggered an arrhythmia. His death from ventricular fibrillation, an erratic and disorganized firing of impulses from the ventricle chambers of the heart, would have occurred within minutes.

While a heart attack is another possible explanation for Presley's death, it is less likely. Presley had only mild to moderate amount of plaque in the coronary vessels and aorta, not substantial enough to have caused significant occlusion of the coronary vessels and blockage of blood flow to the heart.[18] Further, Francisco didn't mention finding evidence of death of cardiac muscle at the autopsy, and Presley never complained of angina or chest pain.[18]

Life and Career

Presley was born in 1935 in Mississippi, but when he was a teenager, his family moved to Memphis, Tennessee.[19] Presley's mother, to whom Presley was very close throughout his life, bought him his first guitar as a present for his eleventh birthday.[20] A few years later, he won the high school's talent show.[20]

Presley first heard gospel music at the Assembly of God Church where he and his parents often prayed.[21] It would become a strong influence in his music. "Since I was two years old, all I knew was gospel music," he said.[21]

After graduating high school, Presley worked as a movie theater usher and truck driver, and in his spare time, he sang locally as the Hillbilly Cat.[21] He auditioned for two local bands but was advised to stick to driving a truck. He would never make it as a singer, he was told.

[22] When he auditioned for a spot on *Arthur Godfrey's Talent Scouts*, he was turned down there as well.[23]

When Sam Phillips, the owner of Sun Studio, heard Presley's first demo record, he immediately signed him to a record label.[23] It wasn't until 1954, when he released "That's All Right," that Presley's singing career began to take off. He appeared several times on *Louisiana Hayride* and released "Heartbreak Hotel" in 1956. It quickly became his first number one hit. He followed "Heartbreak Hotel" with "Blue Suede Shoes" and a self-titled album with a photo of himself playing the guitar on the cover. Then, in April of the same year, Presley appeared on the *Milton Berle Show*, and in July on the *Steve Allen Show*. It was the first time the *Steve Allen Show* topped the *Ed Sullivan Show* in the TV ratings.

Sullivan labeled Presley "unfit for family viewing."[24] He was reluctant to feature Presley on his weekly variety show, fearing Presley's hip-swinging gyrations were so sexually suggestive they would offend the viewership. However, when he saw Allen's ratings, Sullivan relented and booked Presley for three performances, ordering the camera crew to show Presley only from the waist up.[25] Presley's appearances on the *Ed Sullivan Show* shot him to national celebrity status, and his singing of the ballad "Love Me Tender" brought in a million advance orders.

Not everyone was enamored with Presley's singing style. Ben Gross of the *New York Daily News* reviewed one of Presley's performances and wrote he "rotates his pelvis [and] gave an exhibition that was suggestive and vulgar, tinged with the kind of animalism that should be confined to dives and bordellos."[26] Many executives in the music industry thought the way to contend with Presley and his "vulgar" music was to promote a singer whose wholesome American values were beyond reproach. Pat Boone was just such a person. He was married to his high school sweetheart and sang in church and on local television and radio stations.[27] By making rock and roll seem safe and nonthreatening, Boone was the antithesis to Presley.[27]

Presley had ten number one singles by the time he was drafted into the United States Army in 1958. That number would increase to eighteen number one singles and thirty-three appearances in films by the time he died.[28]

RCA was concerned people would forget Presley while he was in the army. To keep his name in the public's mind, the studio released songs he had prerecorded, including "Hard-Headed Woman," "One Night," and "A Food Such as I." When his military duty came to an end in 1960, Presley went back to the studio and recorded

"Stuck on You," "It's Now or Never," and "Are You Lonesome Tonight?" They all became huge hits.

By 1967, Presley's films, although profitable, were generally panned by critics.[29] And while his recordings sold well, many people considered Presley a "has-been."[30] However, on December 3, 1968, Presley's television special, later known as the *Comeback Special*, captured 42 percent of the total television viewership. The unexpected success led to sold-out performances in Las Vegas. *Rolling Stone* magazine called Presley "supernatural, his own resurrection."[31]

In 1970, four days before Christmas, Presley met President Richard Nixon in the White House Oval Office.[32] Two years later, he won a Golden Globe Award for Best Documentary Film for *Elvis on Tour*. The following year, his *Aloha from Hawaii* television special was the first concert by a solo artist to be aired globally.[33]

While in military service, Presley met Priscilla, a fourteen-year-old teenager.[34] They married almost eight years later.[34] By the time they divorced in 1973, Presley was addicted to drugs. His addiction, which began approximately six years prior to his divorce, was aided by Dr. Nichopoulos. "Dr. Nick," as he was known, had been treating Presley for chronic insomnia and supplying him with amphetamines, barbiturates, and narcotics for several years.[34] Presley's face became bloated, and his weight increased, by some estimates close to three hundred and fifty pounds.

Sometime after Presley died, the Tennessee Board of Health filed legal proceedings against Dr. Nick, claiming he had been overprescribing Presley opioids and other medications for many years.[35] However, Dr. Nick was exonerated after he countered that Presley was addicted to drugs and he had tried to keep him away from illegal drugs, often prescribing placebos.[36]

Dr. Nick was indicted by the Shelby County Sheriff in May 1980 for overprescribing drugs not only to Presley but also to Jerry Lee Lewis, another rock and roll singer, as well as to twelve other patients. However, he was acquitted of all these charges as well.[37] Then, in 1995, the Tennessee Board of Medical Examiners finally and permanently suspended Dr. Nick's medical license.[38]

Conclusion

Presley was an unusually good-looking singer with jet-black hair and long sideburns who completely changed the popular music of his time. His rockabilly style of music was unique and a major cultural shift from the music being performed at the time by Frank Sinatra and the Glen Miller Orchestra. The up-tempo fusion of country music and rhythm and blues with a bit of gospel thrown in provided young people the musical outlet they had been craving.[39] Girls screamed whenever he sang, especially when he moved his hips, leading to his nickname, "Elvis the Pelvis."[40] When a receptionist at Sun Studio asked Presley who he sounded like, he replied, "I don't sound like nobody."[41]

John Lennon of the Beatles acknowledged that without Presley, there wouldn't have been the Beatles.[42] Presley "is probably the most important star of all time," said acclaimed journalist and author Allanna Nash.[42] He "not only changed, but directed the course of both popular music and popular culture of the '50s."[43]

The United States Postal Service issued a memorial Elvis Presley stamp in 1993.[44] It became the top-selling commemorative postage stamp of all time.[44]

Even today, Presley's popularity has never been greater. Millions of fans buy his music every year.[45] More than five hundred thousand people visit Presley's Graceland mansion annually, with 50 percent of the visitors under the age of thirty-five.[46]

In 2019, Presley was ranked second to Michael Jackson on Forbes' list of the Top-Earning Dead Celebrities.[46] In the same year, his estate earned $39 million.[47]

According to one report, which cites data from the United States Internal Revenue Service, there are currently more than eighty-four thousand Elvis Presley impersonators in the United States.[48]

Presley "was so unique, his influence can still be felt years later in music, culture, dress, hairstyles, and pop stardom," Nash said.[49] "I expect Elvis will still be someone that generations will study long after you and I are in the grave … He's probably the most influential figure in the twentieth century."

CHAPTER 7

Natalie Wood

Died November 29, 1981

IN THE FALL of 1981, Natalie Wood, a talented actress who was once voted "The Most Beautiful Teenager in the World" by *Life* magazine, began working on what turned out to be her last film.[1] Along with her costar Christopher Walken, the two played an estranged couple, part of a team of high-tech research scientists in the science fiction thriller *Brainstorm*. However, during a break for the Thanksgiving holiday, Wood and her husband, Robert Wagner, went on a sailing trip aboard their sixty-foot yacht, *Splendour*, to Catalina Island, off the southern coast of California, and asked Walken to join them.[2]

At about five o'clock on Saturday evening, November 28, Wood, Wagner, Walken, and Dennis Daven, the captain of the *Splendour*, went ashore to Doug's Harbor Restaurant, where they were seen drinking daiquiris, champagne, and wine.[3] They drank two more bottles of champagne during dinner and appeared intoxicated when they left the restaurant.[4] Don Whiting, the restaurant's night manager, was concerned for their safety, so he called the harbor patrol to make sure the group reached the *Splendour* without incident.[4]

Once they arrived aboard the yacht, Wagner, Walken, and Daven continued to drink in the ship's main cabin, but at around midnight, they discovered that Wood and the inflatable dinghy, a Zodiac called the *Valiant*, were missing.[5] Wood still wasn't in bed at one thirty in the morning. Wagner, now very concerned, got on the ship's radio and reported her missing.[5]

Aboard his boat *Easy Rider*, Paul Miller heard Wagner's voice on the radio's harbor channel.[6] "This is *Splendour*," Wagner said.[7] "We think we may have someone missing in an eleven-foot rubber dinghy." Overhearing the conversation, Whiting, the restaurant manager, radioed one of his friends on the isthmus of Catalina Island and asked him to go to the *Splendour* to assess the situation.[8] A search was begun after it was confirmed that Wood and the dinghy were missing.[9]

A sheriff's helicopter summoned at seven thirty in the morning spotted Wood's body lying facedown in the Pacific Ocean, about two hundred yards off an isolated cove known as Blue Cavern Point.[10] Clad in a blue and red plaid flannel nightgown, argyle woolen socks, and a down-filled red jacket, the body had numerous bruises on the arms and legs and foam coming from the mouth. [10] The dinghy was later found washed up on shore, the ignition key in the off position, the gear in neutral, and the oars tied down, a clear indication the boat had never been used.[10]

Investigators determined Wood left the *Splendour* sometime between 10:45 p.m. and midnight on Saturday night of the Thanksgiving weekend.[11] The time of death was fixed at about midnight, which meant Wood could have been in the water at least an hour and a quarter.[12] The question that came to my mind as I reviewed the records was, how did Wood wind up in the ocean when she was afraid of the water?[13]

The Autopsy

Wood's autopsy was performed by Dr. Joseph H. Choi, a deputy medical examiner of the county of Los Angeles.

He was assisted by Dr. Ronald N. Kornblum and supervised by Dr. Noguchi, the chief medical examiner-coroner.[14] Noguchi had been slowly building a reputation as the "Coroner to the Stars," having already performed or assisted in Monroe's and Joplin's autopsies.[15] His high-profile tenure would be filled with accusations of using his office for personal gain, claims he fought until he was demoted in 1982 for mismanaging his office and sensationalizing the deaths of celebrities.[15]

Wood's head had no scalp or skull fractures, so it was unlikely her death was due to a concussion.[16] Also, there was no evidence of strangulation.[16] I was taken aback, however, when I saw how many fresh bruises were on Wood's arms and legs, as well as the number of abrasions on the left side of her face.[16] Choi concluded that most of the bruises were probably sustained when Wood drowned.[16]

After I reviewed the records, I was confident Wood's death was the result of drowning. There was froth coming out of her mouth and nostrils, a clear sign of drowning, and her lungs were heavy and filled with watery fluid and froth, as were other parts of her respiratory system—larynx, trachea, and bronchi.[16] In addition, a large amount of magnesium and chloride was detected in blood collected from the left side of Wood's heart compared to the right.[16] This has previously been reported in people who aspirated water and drowned.[17]

When I looked for evidence in the autopsy report of other possible causes of Wood's death, I didn't find any. Although there was 30 percent narrowing of one of her descending coronary arteries and mild atherosclerosis in her aorta, these were not sufficiently severe to have caused a heart attack.[18] Also, the heart was of normal size and weight and wasn't a risk factor for sudden death. Wood's brain had some mild to moderate congestion, but it wasn't of any toxicological significance.[18] Furthermore, the liver was of normal appearance and color, with no evidence of cirrhosis or fatty degeneration.[18]

Cause and Manner of Death

Alcohol was detected in Wood's blood, the concentration of which was 75 percent above the current legal limit for drivers in the United States.[18] Based on my calculations, Wood's blood alcohol level would have been nearly twice the current legal limit when she was still on the *Splendour*. With that much alcohol in her system, she would have been fatigued and would have had difficulty maintaining her balance. Also, her judgment would have been significantly impaired.[19]

Besides caffeine and alcohol, the only drugs detected in Wood's blood were low, therapeutic amounts of propoxyphene, an opioid painkiller, and cyclizine, an antinausea medication. Both drugs have similar side effects, including drowsiness, sedation, and dizziness. When taken along with alcohol, the two medications would have enhanced alcohol's sedative properties and its ability to cause unsteadiness.

The public was skeptical when Noguchi announced that, in his opinion, Wood's death was an accidental drowning. Most everyone agreed Wood drowned in the Pacific Ocean. However, many refused to believe her death was an accident. More likely, they thought, she was murdered by her husband, Robert Wagner. Fueling the mystery further was the fact that the events surrounding Wood's death had all the elements of intrigue—a beautiful young woman, a handsome husband, and an equally handsome male guest aboard a sixty-foot yacht, as well as lots of drinking of alcohol, and a suspicious drowning in the middle of the night while on a Thanksgiving holiday.

Thirty years after Wood's body was discovered floating in the ocean, the Los Angeles County Sheriff's Department reopened the investigation. Dr. Lakshmanan Sathyavagiswaran, the new chief medical examiner-coroner, was asked to reevaluate the case and to provide his opinions in a supplemental report.[20]

Sathyavagiswaran interviewed Noguchi, but he was unable to speak with Choi, who had already died.[21] After reviewing the relevant records, Sathyavagiswaran concluded that because of the jewelry and clothing Wood wore the night she died, her intoxicated state, the lack of a life jacket, the fact the dinghy was never used, Wood's urine-filled bladder, the lack of a suicide note, and the fact that the drowning occurred in darkness, he couldn't exclude the possibility that Wood's entry into the water was unplanned.[21] He further reported that the location and multiplicity of the bruises, the lack of head trauma and facial bruising, and the freshness of the bruises supported his opinion the bruising could have occurred on the *Splendour*, before Wood entered the water.[21] Sathyavagiswaran agreed, however, based on the presence of partially digested food in Wood's stomach, that the time of death was approximately midnight. But he noted there were conflicting statements made as to when Wood went missing and whether there were verbal arguments between her and Wagner the night she died.[22]

"The cause of death will be changed [from drowning] to drowning 'and other undetermined factors,'" Sathyavagiswaran announced after he submitted his supplemental report, and the "manner [of death] will be changed [from accidental] to undetermined."[23]

The question that gnawed at me after I reviewed the supplemental report was why Sathyavagiswaran qualified Wood's death by adding the phrase "and other undetermined factors." Was it because of political pressure to justify opening a new police investigation? And what other factors did he have in mind? Certainly hypothermia was a possibility, as well as the presence of alcohol, propoxyphene, and cyclizine in Wood's blood, but neither he nor Noguchi mentioned these as contributing factors in Wood's death in their reports.[24] As for Wood's bruises, they weren't life threatening, and she didn't suffer from an infection or have significant anatomical abnormalities that could have caused her death.[24]

According to Paola Crespo of the *Huff Post*, who excerpted portions of Noguchi's book *Coroner*, Noguchi thought alcohol had played a significant role in Wood's death, but one of his staff dissuaded him from mentioning it.[25] In his book, Noguchi amplified on his theory, claiming that Wood must have lost her balance when she untied the dinghy and had fallen into the water, and her bruises were sustained when she attempted to board the dinghy.[25] He further claimed the heavy weight of her water-logged jacket had dragged her into the ocean and had exhausted her energy. With that much alcohol in her blood, Wood couldn't have been thinking clearly, Noguchi said, which was the reason she didn't take off her jacket.[25] As hypothermia set in, she lost consciousness and drowned.[25] Some might say it was a plausible explanation for Wood's death. However, its main elements, hypothermia and alcohol, were not mentioned as contributing factors in her death, either in Noguchi's or Sathyavagiswaran's final reports.

Life and Career

Wood began her film career when she was just four years old, appearing for fifteen seconds in the 1943 film *Happy Land* and three years later in *Tomorrow Is Forever*.[26] Her big break, and the role that made her a child star, occurred in 1947 when she was cast as the little girl who doubted the existence of Santa Claus in *Miracle on 34th Street*.[27] The public loved Wood in the film, and it soon became a Christmas classic.[28] Throughout the 1940s and early 1950s, Wood acted in at least sixteen more films.[28] "I spent practically all my time [as a child actor] in the company of adults," Wood said.[28] "I was very withdrawn, very shy, and I did what I was told."[28]

When she was sixteen, Wood's superb performance as a rebellious teenager in *Rebel without a Cause* earned her an Oscar nomination for Best Supporting Actress.[29] In her next film, *The Searchers*, a Western classic, she played a Caucasian teenage girl who was kidnapped by Indians.[30] But by the early 1960s, Wood was ready to tackle adult roles.

Wood played "Deanie" Loomis to Warren Beatty's Bud Stamper in the 1961 film *Splendor in the Grass*, a dramatic movie of a teenage girl dealing with repressed sexual desires. Her performance earned her nominations for an Academy Award and a Golden Globe Award.[31] Her next acting assignment was as Maria in *West Side Story*, a modern-day version of *Romeo and Juliet*. The film about two young people in rival gangs in New York City who fall in love won ten Oscars, including Best Picture. When Wood sang, "Hold my hand and we're halfway there …" I thought she was singing just for me. It was only later I learned that even though she could sing, Wood's voice was dubbed because it wasn't considered strong enough.[32]

Wood won her third Oscar nomination for her performance in *Love with the Proper Stranger*.[33] After a three-year break, she acted in another hit movie, *Bob & Carol & Ted & Alice*. Television appearances soon followed, including in shows such as *The Affair*, *Cat on a Hot Tin Roof*, *Switch*, and on *Hart to Hart* with Wagner.[33]

In 1957, when she was only nineteen years old, Wood married Wagner. She would later admit she fell in love with him when she was just ten.[33] "We loved each other tremendously," she said after their divorce became final.[34] "It was disillusioning when it didn't work out." However in 1972, just three months after she divorced her second husband, Wood again married Wagner.[35] "Sometimes, it's better to have the devil you know than the devil you don't," she said after she married Wagner for the second time.[36] Little did she know what lay ahead.

Conclusion

Five years after Sathyavagiswaran issued his supplemental report, Lieutenant John Corina of the Los Angeles County Sheriff's Department announced that Wood's death was "suspicious."[37] "We're closer to understanding what happened," he told reporters.[38] "As we've investigated the case over the last six years, I think [Wagner] is more of a person of interest now. She got in the water somehow, and I don't think she got in the water by herself."[39] Ralph Hernandez, an investigator in the case, concurred. "We have not been able to prove this was a homicide," he said. "And we haven't been able to prove that this was an accident either."[40]

Wood's sister, Lana, had a different opinion. "I believe that there was a horrible fight onboard the *Splendour*. I think it escalated to a point where she was either struck or pushed. I don't believe that it was planned. I cannot ever believe that [Wagner] had purposefully done something to hurt her."[41]

Walken summed it up best when he said, "The people who are convinced that there was something more to it than what came out in the investigation will never be satisfied with the truth. Because the truth is, there is nothing more to it. It was an accident."[42]

Nearly forty years after Wood's death, the mystery of how she died continues to be controversial. Much of the evidence in the case has been discarded, Wagner is almost in his tenth decade, and several of the principal participants in the case have either died or have retired. [43] Nevertheless, considering the public's fascination with the circumstances surrounding Wood's death, I doubt we have heard the final word in this mysterious drowning.

In 1977, Billy Joel, the American singer-songwriter, penned "Only the Good Die Young."[44] The song could have easily been written about Natalie Wood.

CHAPTER 8

John Belushi

Died March 5, 1982

THE CHATEAU MARMONT Hotel in West Hollywood was a place where many celebrities had stayed in the past.[1] John Belushi, a well-known comedian who had appeared on *Saturday Night Live*, resided there in early March 1982, during which time he spent about $2,500 a week on drugs. [2] On March 1, he and his female companion, Cathy Evelyn Smith, spent their time together injecting cocaine and drinking wine, but on Thursday evening, March 4, they went to Rock City, a private club where drugs were not allowed.[2] Belushi was drinking so heavily that night that he and Smith left the club at one o'clock in the morning.[3] When they arrived at their hotel, Belushi had to be helped to his room. After vomiting in the bathroom, he resumed drinking wine and injecting more cocaine.[3]

At six thirty on Friday morning, Belushi took a shower and then went back to bed, shaking and wheezing. [4] When his physical therapist visited him at twelve thirty in the afternoon, he found Belushi still in bed and unresponsive, with a large amount of mucus in his nose. He pulled Belushi onto the carpet and called paramedics, who pronounced Belushi dead fifteen minutes later.[4] He was thirty-three years old.

Dr. Noguchi, the chief medical examiner-coroner of the county of Los Angeles, and several members of his medical staff arrived at the Chateau Marmont to investigate. They found traces of a white powder, two folded papers, a green leafy substance in a plastic container, cigarette papers, and a prescription bottle containing two tablets of Actifed, a combination of the antihistamine, tripolidine, and the decongestant, pseudoephedrine, that Belushi had been taking for his sinus condition.[5] All of these items were collected as evidence for further analysis.[5]

Police questioned Smith the night Belushi died, but she was released. However, when she was interviewed by the *National Enquirer*, Smith admitted she had been supplying and administering "speedballs" to Belushi, a combination of cocaine, a stimulant, and heroin, a depressant. After her interview, police charged Smith with murder and drug-related offenses.[6]

The Autopsy

Belushi's autopsy was conducted in Los Angeles, a city that was quickly becoming the epicenter of celebrity autopsies.[7] It was clear to Dr. Kornblum, the deputy medical examiner of the county of Los Angeles who performed the autopsy, that at five feet eight inches tall and weighing 222 pounds, Belushi was obese and in poor physical condition before he died.[7]

Kornblum had assisted in Natalie Wood's autopsy. By the time he resigned from the medical examiner-coroner's office in 1990, he would perform the autopsy on the bodies of several other celebrities, including William Holden and Truman Capote.[8]

An external examination revealed that Belushi's nasal septum, the dividing wall that separates the two nasal cavities, was intact, suggesting Belushi's well-documented chronic illicit drug use probably occurred more often by injection than by nasal insufflation.[9]

After performing the midline incision and exposing the internal organs, Kornblum identified the liver, which was congested, the spleen, which was enlarged and congested, the urinary bladder and lungs, both of which were distended, and the heart, whose weight was above normal, mainly because both ventricle chambers were mildly enlarged.[9] However, the valves separating the heart chambers were functioning normally.[9] And while the coronary arteries and aorta had mild atherosclerotic plaque, these were not severe enough to have caused a heart attack.[9] Also, it's unlikely Belushi's death was caused by an arrhythmia since he had a low risk for sudden death.

Large amount of air was trapped in the alveoli, tiny air sacs in the lungs that allowed for the rapid exchange of gas.[9] And while Belushi's brain was swollen, there was no evidence of hemorrhage, injury, or disease, the most common causes of brain swelling.[9] Neither were there fractures in the skull, another potential cause of the accumulated fluid.[9] This suggested that the brain swelling was probably due to chronic use of illicit drugs, another potential cause of fluid accumulation in the brain.

As for the remaining organs, the prostate was normal, both kidneys were of the expected weight, and the pituitary, thyroid, and adrenal glands were all unremarkable.[9]

Cause and Manner of Death

The cause of Belushi's death became apparent when multiple fresh needle marks were found on both of his arms and a small amount of foamy pink fluid was detected in his upper airways and oral and nasal cavities, findings consistent with an opioid overdose.[9] When high levels of morphine, the active metabolite of heroin, and free, unmetabolized cocaine were detected in Belushi's blood, it confirmed he died from an overdose of a speedball.[9] Belushi had probably taken the heroin and cocaine mixture not long before he died because not enough time had passed for the cocaine to be completely metabolized.

Undoubtedly, the stimulating effects of cocaine wore off much sooner than the central nervous system depressant effects of heroin. The delayed effects of heroin led to death from respiratory depression.[9] The manner of death was an accident.

Life and Career

Growing up in Chicago, Belushi attended the University of Wisconsin and the College of DuPage.[10] After acting in summer stock and in the West Compass Players, an improvisational comedy troupe modeled after Chicago's Second City, he joined Second City and then the cast of

National Lampoon's Lemmings, an off Broadway rock musical revue.[10] His career took off in 1975 after he joined *Saturday Night Live*, the highly successful late-night television show, where his manic and zany style of comedy blossomed.[10]

Following his stint on *Saturday Night Live*, Belushi acted in two films—*National Lampoon's Animal House* and *The Blues Brothers*. Throughout this period, he experimented with drugs—marijuana, LSD, and amphetamines—but it was during the early to mid-1970s that his drug use escalated and he became addicted to cocaine.[11]

Belushi's boundless energy was reminiscent of Robin Williams. However, the two comedians were completely different. Williams was a bundle of kinetic energy, always in motion, whereas Belushi's energy was best reflected in his rapidly evolving mind as he constantly wondered how to best milk the next comedic moment. Perfect examples of his genius were his classic imitations of a samurai and of the rock and roll singer Joe Cocker.

John Landis, the director of *National Lampoon's Animal House*, remembered Belushi this way: "He was strong like a tractor and smart like a bull and he really could have gone on to do anything."[12] Unfortunately, it was not to be.

Conclusion

"We had a budget in for cocaine for night shoots," Dan Aykroyd, Belushi's costar in *The Blues Brothers* told *Vanity Fair* in 2012.[13] "John, he just loved what it did. It sort of brought him alive at night."[13]

Aside from the obvious health problems associated with using illicit drugs, it is impossible to know precisely what one is receiving when purchasing illegal drugs. Heroin is often cut with fentanyl, talc, or other pharmaceuticals with little, if any, accuracy in measuring or dosing. This can lead to unexpected side effects, including death. And when the route of exposure is by intravenous injection, as was the case in Belushi, the effects occur rapidly, providing very little time for medical intervention.

CHAPTER 9

Karen Carpenter

Died February 4, 1983

On February 4, 1983, Karen Carpenter, the female singer of the highly successful brother-sister team, the Carpenters, was visiting her parents in Downey, California. When her mother entered the kitchen at about 8:50 in the morning, she found Carpenter lying unresponsive on the floor.[1] Paramedics soon arrived and initiated CPR. Carpenter was then transported to Downey Community Hospital, where laboratory tests showed that her blood sugar level was ten times higher than normal. [2] Efforts to resuscitate Carpenter failed, and death from "hyperosmolar coma," a condition characterized by a severe high blood sugar level and dehydration, was pronounced at 9:51 a.m.[3] She was thirty-two years old.[3]

The Autopsy

Dr. Kornblum became the acting chief medical examiner-coroner of the county of Los Angeles in 1982. As deputy medical examiner, he had performed autopsies on the bodies of Natalie Wood and John Belushi. Now, lying on the gurney in the autopsy room was the body of another celebrity, an all too young female whose face he instantly recognized.

Carpenter's autopsy began at two thirty in the afternoon, about five and a half hours after she died.[3] There was no evidence her death was due to foul play, nor that it was caused by a concussion, as if from a fall. The head was free of injury and skull fractures, and the brain had no hemorrhage.[3] Furthermore, there were no injuries to the neck or legs, nor any sign of disease.[3]

On external examination, Carpenter's body was remarkably thin, as were the arms. Measuring sixty-four inches long, Carpenter weighed only 108 pounds.[3]

Carpenter's abdomen, small bowel, and colon were all distended, a finding for which there were several possible explanations.[3] While there was some evidence of respiratory congestion, with a pink, foamy fluid in the airways as well as in the lungs, there was no noticeable aspiration of food particles or pneumonia.[3]

The spleen, as well as the liver and its associated lymph node, were enlarged, but the weight of both organs was within the normal range.[3] The brain, pancreas, musculoskeletal system, kidneys, and bladder were all unremarkable and free of traumatic injury, lesions, or tumors.[3]

What was most surprising was the unusual appearance of the cardiovascular system. The heart was normal in shape and configuration, but it was conspicuously small, weighing only 60 percent of the average female heart.[3] The low body weight and the small heart size were consistent with Carpenter's history of having suffered from anorexia nervosa, a debilitating eating disorder.[3] Nevertheless, the valves separating the heart chambers were anatomically normal, and the coronary and pulmonary arteries, as well as the aorta, had minimal atherosclerotic plaque.[3]

Interestingly, Carpenter's stomach contained about two ounces of a dark green, dry, and hydrous material whose consistency was of dried tea leaves.[3] The duodenum, present between the stomach and the small bowel, also had a soft, semiliquid yellowish-green material, as did the small bowel and colon.[3] The description of these materials in the digestive tract is consistent with cascara and emetine-containing ipecac leaves, two over-the-counter laxatives that were popular at the time. That may explain why the abdomen, small bowel, and colon were distended and why Carpenter's body was dehydrated. Notably absent from the stomach was any identifiable food or pill fragments.[3]

Cause and Manner of Death

Carpenter's obsession with her weight began after she graduated high school.[4] Always referred to as "chubby" and weighing 145 pounds, Carpenter went on the Stillman diet, a low-carb high-protein diet that in 1967 was all the rage.[5] The diet allowed for six meals and eight glasses of water per day and promised weight loss of many pounds in just a few weeks. In fact, Carpenter lost twenty-five pounds within six months.[6] Despite the difficulty of trying to eat a healthy diet and constantly being on the road, Carpenter was able to maintain her new weight for six years.[7]

Sometime in August 1973, the Carpenters performed at Lake Tahoe, Nevada. Later, Carpenter saw a photo taken of her at the concert that accentuated her midriff.[8] Unhappy with the way she looked, she hired a personal trainer who recommended a low-calorie, high-carbohydrate diet to supplement her exercise routine.

[8] However, instead of losing weight, Carpenter gained muscle, so she decided to fire the trainer and to purchase a hip cycle, portable indoor exercise equipment that helped tone the muscle of the hips.[8] Using the hip cycle every morning, even while touring, Carpenter lost twenty more pounds.[9] "If she'd been able to stop there, then life would have been beautiful," said Carole Curb, sister of Carpenter's boyfriend at the time.[10] "[But] Karen got carried away. She just couldn't stop."[10]

By September 1975, Carpenter's weight had declined to just ninety-one pounds, and she started wearing layers of clothing to disguise how emaciated she had become.[10] "She would start with a long-sleeved shirt and then put a blouse over that," said Sherwin Bash, Carpenter's agent, "and a sweater over that and a jacket over that."[10] Having no energy, Carpenter was forced to take two months off and to cancel shows.

Over the next five years, Carpenter continued to struggle with her weight and eating disorder. By January 1982, she was taking a large number of laxative pills every night and ten thyroid tablets daily to stimulate her metabolism.[11] She began to see Steven Levenkron, a psychotherapist, who specialized in eating disorders, but according to her brother, even after several months of five days per week of private sessions, Levenkron's treatment plan wasn't achieving the desired results.[12]

On September 20, 1982, Carpenter, now weighing about seventy-nine pounds, was admitted to New York's Lenox Hill Hospital to undergo surgery for intravenous feeding, known as hyperalimentation.[13] Within a few days, she gained twelve pounds, ultimately gaining twenty-five pounds.[13] Solid food slowly replaced the intravenous feedings, but by the time Carpenter's brother came to visit his sister a month later, Carpenter still looked extremely emaciated.[14]

One of the most serious complications of an eating disorder such as anorexia nervosa is the potential life-threatening toxic effects on the heart, which occurs in 80 percent of patients who suffer from this condition.[15] "Because of the nutritional problems created by the anorexia nervosa, you get chemical imbalances and that leads to heart irregularities," said Kornblum.[16] Carpenter's "heart stopped," he added.

Based on the autopsy findings, Kornblum concluded that Carpenter died a natural death from "emetine cardiotoxicity" due to anorexia nervosa.[17] Simply stated, Carpenter's death was caused by toxic effects to the heart due to excessive use of laxatives in pursuit of being thin.[17] I found no reason to disagree with Kornblum's opinions.

Life and Career

Born in 1950 in New Haven, Connecticut, Carpenter preferred to play softball, whereas her brother was a musical prodigy.[18] To provide Carpenter's brother a better opportunity to get into the recording industry, the family moved to Downey, a suburb of Los Angeles, when Carpenter was thirteen years old.[18]

In her first year at Downy High School, Carpenter joined the school's marching band, where she played the glockenspiel.[19] When she saw one of her bandmates playing the drums, she took a liking to the instrument.[19] Carpenter's parents saw their daughter's budding interest and bought her a set of drums.[19] Later, after she became famous, Carpenter said she always thought of herself as "a drummer who sang."[20]

At fifteen, Carpenter teamed up with her brother and Wes Jacobs, a tuba and bass player, to form the jazz instrumental group the Richard Carpenter Trio.[21] On June 24, 1966, the trio won "The Battle of the Bands" at the Hollywood Bowl.[21] However, when Jacobs left to enroll at the Julliard School of the Performing Arts, the world's leading music, drama, and dance school in New York City, Carpenter and her brother formed a new band, Spectrum, this time concentrating on Carpenter's contralto vocals, which had since matured.[21] By the time Spectrum disbanded in mid-1968, Carpenter's singing style had fully developed, and her brother's skill for musical arrangements had likewise substantially improved.[21] Together, they formed their new and final group, the Carpenters.[21]

It was by mere coincidence that Herb Alpert, cofounder of A&M Records, heard one of the Carpenters' demo tapes in 1969.[21] "The first note I heard from this tape was Carpenter's voice," Alpert said.[21] "It felt like her voice was on the couch, like she was sitting next to me."[21] Loving the harmonies and the musical arrangements, Alpert immediately offered the Carpenters a recording contract.[21] It was the beginning of what would become a very successful musical career.

The Carpenters' first album, *Offering*, was released in November 1969.[21] It included their special arrangements of the Beatles' 1965 hit "Ticket to Ride."[21] Sung as a ballad in a minor key with beautiful harmonies, one critic claimed it "virtually redefined the song."[21] It was followed by "Close to You," which reached number one on American charts and won a Grammy for Best Contemporary Vocal Performance by a Duo, Group or Chorus, as well as the 1970 Grammy for Best New Artist.[21]

The Carpenters released more hits over the next several years, including "We've Only Just Begun," "For

All We Know," "Rainy Days and Mondays," "Superstar,"
"It's Going to Take Some Time," and "Goodbye to Love."
[21] They performed in live concerts all over the United
States, as well as in Europe and Japan, and had several
television appearances and specials.[21] And in May 1973,
the Carpenters were invited to perform at the White
House in honor of West German Chancellor Willy
Brandt.[21]

In 1980, Carpenter married a divorced real estate
developer who was nine years her senior.[22] After the
wedding, she discovered that her husband had undergone
a vasectomy and refused to have it reversed.[22] The
marriage lasted only fourteen months.[22]

Conclusion

Dr. Richard Morton, a London physician, was the first to
report a case of "nervous consumption" in 1969, which
Dr. William Gull later named "anorexia nervosa."[23]
According to the National Eating Disorders Association,
the eating disorder, 85 percent of which occurs in women,
is characterized by a distorted body image, weight loss,
and difficulty maintaining an appropriate body weight
that corresponds with the height, age, and stature of an
individual.[24] While the exact cause of anorexia nervosa
is unknown, there is some evidence to indicate an

association with genetic, psychological, and sociocultural components.

Although the number of cases of anorexia nervosa had been climbing since the 1950s, it wasn't until Carpenter died in 1982 that the public became aware of this disorder. "Anorexia nervosa was so new that I didn't even know how to pronounce it until 1980," said John Bettis, one of the Carpenters' band members.[25]

Carpenter's death proved that being too thin can be just as deadly as being too heavy. While Carpenter died young from degeneration of the heart caused by anorexia nervosa, Cass Elliot, who was also young when she died, had heart failure brought about by her obesity. In both cases, death was from toxic effects to the heart.

Carpenter's voice will surely be missed for a long time but especially at Christmas, when "Merry Christmas Darling," a song she recorded in 1978 that is nearly as popular as Bing Crosby's "White Christmas," fills the airwaves. Paul McCartney of the Beatles said Carpenter had "the best female voice in the world: melodic, tuneful and distinctive."[26] Elton John called her "one of the greatest voices of our lifetime."[27] Both singers expressed my sentiments entirely.

CHAPTER 10

Sam Kinison

Died April 10, 1992

SUNDAY, APRIL 5, 1992, was a special day. After a five-year relationship, Sam Kinison, a comedian best known for his loud scream and his in-your-face vulgar jokes, and Malika, a twenty-seven-year-old dancer, finally married at the Candlelight Chapel in Las Vegas in front of a small group of their closest friends.[1] Dressed in a tuxedo and a red bow tie, Kinison recited his marital vows, tears of joy streaming down his face.[1] After the ceremony, the newlyweds spent their honeymoon at the Mauna Kea Beach Hotel on the Big Island of Hawaii.[1] They were back in Los Angeles early Friday morning, ready to embark for a scheduled sold-out engagement at the Riverside Resort Hotel and Casino in Laughlin, Nevada, a mere four and a half hours' drive away.[1]

The trip to Laughlin began at midday. Kinison, driving the lead car with his new bride by his side, was followed closely by a van transporting his brother, his personal assistant, and his best friend, Carl LaBove.[1] As they reached Needles, California, at about seven thirty in the evening, only forty minutes from their final destination, a 1974 Chevy pickup truck, filled with beer cans and driven in the opposite direction by a seventeen-year-old boy who had been drinking, swerved into their lane.[2] Kinison slowed his vehicle to approximately fifteen miles per hour, but he couldn't avoid the head-on collision.[3]

"I heard the most horrendous crash," LaBove later said.[3] Kinison, who wasn't wearing a seat belt, hit his head on the windshield.[3] He was found lying between the seats.[3] At first, his friends thought he had suffered only minor injuries, but they quickly realized it was much more serious.[3] CPR was administered at the scene and continued in the ambulance while Kinison was being driven to Needles Desert Communities Hospital, but it was too late.[3] He was pronounced dead at 8:31 p.m.[3] Kinison was thirty-eight years old. Malika, Kinison's bride of only one week, survived the accident, but she was knocked unconscious and had significant injuries.[3]

The Autopsy

Two days after the automobile accident, Kinison's autopsy was conducted at the Jensen Carpentry Mortuary in Needles by Dr. Edward T. Paget.[4] Several years later, Paget would be elected the town's mayor.[4]

Kinison's body was markedly obese.[5] There were several abrasions on the head and left kneecap, a possible skull fracture, and a dislocated neck joint but no other noticeable bone fractures.[5] What was most relevant for the identification of cause of death was the unusually large amount of blood in the abdominal cavity, two liters to be precise.[5] It was consistent with the presence of severe internal injuries, including a significant tear in the aorta, the major artery in the body, as well as several torn blood vessels around the small bowel, which were the source of most of the blood.[5] Kinison's internal injuries were so severe that he probably died within minutes of the accident.

Other findings identified in the autopsy included an enlarged heart, known as cardiomegaly, a liver whose size was about two and a half times greater than normal, probably due to Kinison's chronic use of cocaine, and a horseshoe kidney, a rare finding that occurs when two kidneys fuse together during fetal development and form a U shape, like a horseshoe.[5]

What I found especially interesting were the autopsy findings and toxicology test results that, while unrelated to cause of death, hinted at what may have happened at the time of the accident. For example, a large amount of food particles was found in Kinison's mouth, and partially digested food was found in his stomach.[5] These findings suggest that Kinison was eating while driving and may have been temporarily distracted, just as the collision was about to take place. Also, therapeutic amounts of codeine, an opioid, and two tranquilizers, diazepam and alprazolam, all with central nervous system depressant and sedative properties, were detected in Kinison's blood, as well as an inactive metabolite of cocaine.[5] The combination of the tranquilizers and codeine may have sedated Kinison just enough so that he couldn't respond to the emergency situation in a timely manner.

Cause and Manner of Death

Paget concluded Kinison's death was caused by multiple traumatic injuries sustained in an automobile accident.[5] "Drugs did not contribute to the cause of death," Deputy Coroner Gabriel Morales said when the final autopsy report was released, "(but) we are not saying that he wasn't under the influence [of drugs]."[6] Like Morales, I, too, do not propose that Kinison's death was caused by a drug overdose. However, prescription drugs probably contributed to the accident that ultimately led to Kinison's death.

Life and Career

Born about sixty miles southeast of Mount Rainier, Kinison spent most of his youth in Peoria, Illinois.[7] When he was twelve, his parents divorced.[8] As part of the divorce settlement, Kinison and his younger brother remained with their mother.[8] His two older brothers went to live with their father, a Pentecostal preacher. Later, they followed in their father's footsteps and became ministers.[8]

As a rebellious teenager, Kinison was sent to a religious boarding school, but after leaving school and drifting for a few years, he also decided to become a preacher, just like his brothers.[8] However, after seven years in the ministry, Kinison became disillusioned, and in 1977, he told his family he wanted to try his hand as a stand-up comedian instead.[9] Needless to say, his family was skeptical, but Kinison reminded them how he made people laugh in church and "If you can make people laugh in church, you can make them laugh anywhere."

Eventually, the family gave Kinison its blessing, and he moved to Houston, Texas, where he took a workshop in comedy.[10] Within two years, he became one of Houston's top comedians and was featured at the Comedy Annex.[11] Rodney Dangerfield, best known for the catchphrase "I don't get no respect," saw Kinison's act and urged him to continue to develop his talent.[12]

Kinison was twice named the funniest man in Texas by the *Dallas Morning News*, but in 1980, he decided to move to Los Angeles to further hone his craft.[13] He got his big break when Dangerfield showcased him in the *Rodney Dangerfield's Ninth Annual Young Comedians Special* on HBO.[13] Stephen Holden of the *New York Times* heard Kinison's legendary scream and declared, "Mr. Kinison specializes in a grotesque animalist howl that might be described as the primal scream of the married man."[14] David Handelman of *Rolling Stone* magazine called the scream "a supersonic boom born of bile."[15]

On November 14, 1985, *The Tonight Show with David Letterman* featured Kinison in his debut performance as a new and unusual up-and-coming comedian.[15] "We're in for something now, folks," Letterman told the audience.[16] "My next guest is making his television debut tonight, and we believe it's long overdue. He is one of the strangest and most original comedians working today.

Brace yourselves. I'm not kidding. Please welcome— Sam Kinison."[16]

Dressed in a full-length, dark gray overcoat that originally belonged to Richard Widmark, the actor, with his hair neatly hanging long on both sides of his head, Kinison grabbed the microphone and began to pace the floor.[17] "There's still time to call the church and call this off," he told the audience. Some clapped politely, but most hesitated, their nervous laughter barely audible. "I know a lot of you come here, watch TV, wait every night for somebody to come and give you an answer for your lives," Kinison began again. It didn't take long before he went into a loud, screaming tirade about salvation, like the Pentecostal preacher he was before he became a comedian.[17] And then, just when he reached the height of his scream, Kinison's voice became unexpectedly calm. "But I'm not the guy," he said. The audience roared. Now more relaxed, everyone leaned back in his or her chair, laughing and clapping loudly, but Kinison wasn't finished yet. Climbing down from the stage, he approached a man in the audience who sat in the third row. "What's your name?" Kinison asked. "Lou," the man replied. "Lou?" Pause. Only six inches away from the man's face, Kinison screamed, "Ahhhhhhhh! Ahhhhhhhh!" The audience was hysterical.[17]

By 1987, Kinison had been on *Saturday Night Live* and on *Late Night with David Letterman*.[18] He released a successful comedy album, *Louder Than Hell*, and had his first HBO special, *Breaking the Rules*.[18] His first Grammy nomination was in 1988 for his comedy album *You Seen Me Lately?*[18]

Kinison's 1989 appearance on *The Tonight Show with Johnny Carson* caught everyone by surprise.[19] There he was again in his signature overcoat, singing in an unexpectedly beautiful voice the Elvis Presley classic "Are You Lonesome Tonight," backed by a chorus of three male singers.[19] Suddenly, after singing the first verse, Kinison went on a long, loud, rant about love, marriage, and breakup that included an excruciating scream and then calmly ended with "But I'd rather go on hearing your lies. I won't live without you. That's how sick I am."[19] The audience cheered.

"That really brings a tear to your eyes," Carson joked when Kinison sat down on the chair next to him. "That's what love is all about."[19]

I wasn't a fan of Kinison. and apparently, I wasn't the only one. Many thought his humor was downright offensive.[20] I was raised on the masters—Bob Hope, Jack Benny, Groucho Marks. Benny had the audience roaring with laughter just by staring at them with soulful eyes whenever the word *money* was mentioned. That was more than comedy. It was art!

Kinison liked to socialize with the rock and roll crowd and even appeared on the cover of *Rolling Stone* magazine. [21] He had numerous sexual liaisons, including one with his fiancée's younger sister. [22] "Sam lived a lifestyle that was pretty promiscuous," his brother once said. [23] According to published reports, it was only after Kinison died that DNA analysis would reveal that the child for whom LaBove had been paying child support for more than thirteen years was actually fathered by Kinison. [24]

Conclusion

"Every generation has someone who steps outside the norm and offers a voice for the unspeakable attitudes of that time," Kinison once said. "I represent everything that's supposed to be wrong, everything that's forbidden." [25] It was as good an explanation as any for his type of comedy.

There's no doubt that Kinison had his excesses— alcohol, drugs, women, sex. [26] He had also developed an addiction to cocaine. [26] Once, he joked that his cocaine use was so heavy he used a garden hose to inhale. [26] "I've always done drugs," Kinison told Joan Rivers in one of his rare candid interviews. [27] His brother, who was also his manager, remembered, "He had an addictive personality. When he started drinking, he had to drink all the time; when he started doing cocaine, he didn't do a little bit. He had to be there until all the coke was gone."[28]

A one of a kind slash-and-burn comedian, Kinison had a potty mouth. His "comedy of hate" routines incited riots and angered the LGBT community, but his marketing instincts and outrageous behavior sold out large venues.[29]

As a former Pentecostal preacher, Kinison built his entire career by telling jokes about sex and God.[30] "Comedy's fun, people laugh, but I don't know if that makes them feel good about themselves," he said.[31] "Let me put it this way. You can make 'em laugh, but you can't make 'em happy. It takes God to do that."[31]

Richard Belzer, one of Kinison's closest friends, described Kinison this way:[32] "Beneath the rebel was a man with a real heart who had something to say about religion and politics."

At the scene of his automobile accident, Kinison's last words were "Why now? I don't want to die. Why?" as if he was speaking to the Angel of Death.[32] "Okay, okay, okay," he said after a momentary pause and then took his final breath. Was this God's way of calling his preacher son back home, to preach to the choir in his singular way, back to where he belonged?

CHAPTER 11

River Phoenix

Died October 31, 1993

ON THE EVENING of October 30, 1993, during a break in filming of *Dark Blood*, River Phoenix, a popular young actor, went along with his brother Joaquin, his sister Rain, and his girlfriend, Samantha Mathis, to the Viper Room, an exclusive nightclub on the Sunset Strip in West Hollywood.[1] Phoenix was in the bathroom of the club at about one o'clock in the morning when one of his drug dealer friends offered him pure-grade heroin.[2] Almost immediately after he snorted the drug, Phoenix began to shake violently, so one of his friends gave him diazepam, a tranquilizer, to calm him down.[3] Phoenix went back inside the club but soon began to complain he couldn't breathe.[3] When he was helped outside and laid on the sidewalk, he began to have seizures.[3] Joaquin called 911 while Rain and Mathis tried to help Phoenix.[4]

By the time paramedics arrived, Phoenix was already in cardiac arrest.[5] Efforts to resuscitate him failed, and he was transported by ambulance to Cedar-Sinai Medical Center in Los Angeles, where he was pronounced dead.[6] He was only twenty-three years old.[7]

The Autopsy

According to police, foul play was not suspected in Phoenix's death.[8] Also, there was no evidence Phoenix had intended to commit suicide. "The body is identified by toe tags," Dr. Christopher Rogers, the chief of the forensic medicine division of the county of Los Angeles who conducted the autopsy, wrote in the autopsy report, something he had done too many times before.[8]

Phoenix's body was muscular, well built, and without tattoos or abnormal skin discolorations.[8] But what was particularly relevant was the intact, uninflamed nasal septum, just like in John Belushi.[8] The absence of a perforated septum suggested that Phoenix probably wasn't a chronic abuser of illicit drugs by nasal insufflation. However, unlike Belushi, who had multiple fresh needle marks on both of his arms, there were no needle tracks on Phoenix's arms and neck. This supported the notion that Phoenix was probably only an occasional user of illicit drugs.[8]

There were small abrasions on the knuckles of Phoenix's right index finger, and the right thumb and his right shin had a red-purple contusion.[8] However, there was no evidence that Phoenix sustained these bruises in an altercation on the night he died.

The autopsy did not identify any anatomical abnormalities that would have caused Phoenix's death.[8] There were no rib fractures present and no evidence of injury to the chest or abdominal walls.[8] Also, the lungs were free of clots, the heart was of normal weight and configuration and without atherosclerotic plaque, and no hemorrhage was identified in the brain.[8] And when the digestive and endocrine systems, as well as the liver, spleen, kidneys, bladder, and prostate were examined, they were all normal.[8] In addition, no pill fragments were found in the stomach.[8] Without significant anatomical changes to explain why Phoenix died, I turned my attention to the toxicology report.

Cause and Manner of Death

Toxicology analysis detected morphine, the active metabolite of heroin, in Phoenix's blood, as well as a large amount of free, unmetabolized cocaine and its major metabolite.[8] This was a clear indication that, like John Belushi before him, Phoenix had taken a speedball, a combination of cocaine and heroin. He must have consumed the mixture of drugs not long before he died because not enough time had passed for cocaine to have been completely metabolized.[8] And as expected, diazepam was also found in Phoenix's blood, as well as codeine, an opioid medication prescribed for cough, and two over-the-counter nasal decongestants—ephedrine and pseudoephedrine.[8]

A trace of the inactive metabolite of marijuana was found in Phoenix's urine, but unmetabolized marijuana was not detected either in his blood or in his urine.[8] This indicated that Phoenix must have consumed marijuana several hours prior to his death, providing sufficient time for the drug to be completely metabolized and to begin being excreted from his body.[8]

After I reviewed the autopsy and toxicology reports, I agreed with Rogers's conclusion that Phoenix died from acute drug intoxication caused by ingestion of a speedball and that the manner of death was an accident. Other contributing factors in his death included diazepam, ephedrine, and pseudoephedrine, three drugs that can cause an irregular heartbeat and high blood pressure when combined with cocaine and codeine.[9]

"Hopefully it's a wake-up call to the world," Susan Patricola, a spokeswoman for the Phoenix family, said when the autopsy report was released.[10]

Life and Career

The 1986 film *Stand by Me* was memorable for many reasons.[11] First, there was the haunting theme song of the same name, as originally sung by Ben E. King, that accompanied the closing credits. Then, there was the director, Rob Reiner, who played "Meathead," the name Archie Bunker called his son-in-law in the highly controversial television sitcom *All in the Family.*[12] Reiner was an actor and a comedian. *Stand by Me* was only his second film as a director, but he was obviously very talented because he was nominated for a Golden Globe Award for his directorial efforts.[13]

What set *Stand by Me* apart from other films of the day, besides the plot about four youths in Castle Rock, a small town in Oregon, who went looking for the body of a missing boy, was the superb performances by the four young actors who would all go on to achieve great success in the film industry.[14] At sixteen years old, Phoenix was four years older than the other boys.

Phoenix had already accumulated substantial acting experience in television commercials and sitcoms and in his debut film, *Explorers*, before he was selected to act in *Stand by Me*.[15] After *Stand by Me*, he went on to acting roles in *The Mosquito Coast* and *Running on Empty*, for which he was nominated for an Academy Award for Best Supporting Actor, as well as in *Indiana Jones and the Last Crusade*, *My Own Private Idaho*, in which he played a gay hustler, and in *Silent Tongue*.

In the days leading up to his death, Phoenix reportedly was on a drug binge.[16] "I knew he was high that night," his girlfriend, Mathis, told a reporter of the *Irish Times*, "but the heroin that killed him didn't happen until he was in the Viper Room."[17] Bob Forrest, a friend of Phoenix who was also at the Viper Room the night Phoenix died said, that as soon as Phoenix arrived, drugs were passed around.[18] "River was obviously wasted," Forrest wrote in *Running with Monsters*.[18]

Conclusion

Phoenix was a strict vegetarian, an environmentalist, and a member of People for the Ethical Treatment of Animals.[19] He loved music, singing, and playing guitar in his band *Aleka's Attic*.[19] "I think if River was still here, I think he'd be acting, directing, saving the environment, just living and hanging out," said Mathis.[20] But it was not to be.

"How many other beautiful young souls, who remain anonymous to us, have died by using drugs recreationally," Phoenix's mother wrote after her son's death.[21] "It is my prayer that River's leaving in this way will focus the attention of the world on how painfully the spirits of his generation are being worn down."[21]

Some in the film industry compared Phoenix to James Dean, an actor of a bygone era who, like Phoenix, also died young. But like with Dean, other young actors, including Tom Cruise and Leonardo DiCaprio, quickly filled the void left by the death of River Phoenix.[22]

CHAPTER 12

JonBenét Ramsey

Died December 25, 1996

SOMETIME ON CHRISTMAS night in 1996, John and Patsy Ramsey and their two children, JonBenét and her nine-year-old brother, Burke, attended a party at the home of one of their friends.[1] After they returned to their stately, seven-thousand-square-foot residence, JonBenét and her brother were put to bed in their respective second-floor bedrooms.[2] Soon thereafter, John and Patsy retired for the night in their third-floor bedroom, anticipating an early rise to catch a flight to Michigan for a family vacation.[2] Unfortunately, they failed to turn on the security alarm before they went to bed.[3] In addition, a door and seven windows, several of which were accessible from the ground level, were found open the following morning.[3]

At five thirty in the morning, the Ramseys awoke and began to get ready for their trip.[3] While John Ramsey showered, Patsy Ramsey walked down the back spiral staircase to the first level.[3] When she reached the bottom of the stairs, she found a three-page handwritten ransom note.[4] It stated that JonBenét had been kidnapped and demanded $118,000 in exchange for her safe return. [4] After looking in JonBenét's bedroom and finding it empty, Patsy Ramsey checked on Burke and found him sound asleep.[5] Filled with dread, she called the police, despite having been forewarned not to do so, as well as several family friends who came over to provide moral support.[5]

Police arrived at the Ramsey home shortly before 6:00 a.m.[5] Initially, they treated the incident as a kidnapping case. Instead of sealing off the entire residence per usual protocol, they only cordoned off JonBenét's bedroom.[6] As a result, friends and family roamed freely throughout the house, potentially disturbing key evidence.[6]

At about ten o'clock, John Ramsey began to search the basement.[7] He found a partially open window, below which lay a suitcase, which seemed odd since the suitcase was not in its usual storage place.[7] He returned upstairs where everyone had gathered, but sometime in the afternoon, at the suggestion of the police, John Ramsey and one of his friends went back to the basement.[7] The two men searched a playroom and a shower stall and then examined a closet, in front of which was a heavy fireplace grate.[7] Finding nothing unusual, they next set their sights on the wine cellar, which was used as a storage room.[7] Entering the wine cellar first, John turned on the light and discovered his daughter's body.[7] "Oh my God, my baby," he cried out.[7]

Covered with a light-colored blanket, JonBenét had black duct tape over her mouth.[7] Her hands were bound above her head, and a cord attached to a garrote was around her neck.[7] The garrote had a wooden handle made from a paintbrush that was later found in a paint tray in the boiler room.[7] A nylon cord was tied to one end of the handle and a loop with a slipknot, through which JonBenét's neck protruded, was tied to the other.[7] JonBenét's nightgown lay on the floor, nearby.[7]

John Ramsey removed the tape from his daughter's mouth and tried to untie her hands.[7] He picked up her body and brought it upstairs, disturbing the crime scene in the process.[8] Laying JonBenét's body on the living room floor, John Ramsey covered his daughter with a blanket and a sweatshirt.[9] It was only then that police properly secured the entire Ramsey residence and labeled it a crime scene.[10]

The Autopsy

JonBenét's autopsy began at 8:15, the morning of December 27.[11] It was conducted in Boulder, Colorado, by Dr. John E. Meyer, a pathologist in the office of the Boulder County Coroner.[11] Undoubtedly, it was emotionally trying for Meyer to perform an autopsy on the body of such a young child.[11]

"The decedent is clothed in a long sleeved white knit collarless shirt, the mid-anterior chest area of which contains an embroidered silver star decorated with silver sequins," Meyer wrote in the autopsy report.[11] A gold chain with a charm in the form of a cross was wrapped around the neck.[11] The long, white, urine-stained underwear had several red spots consistent with blood.[11] On the shirt's right sleeve was a dried, brown-to-tan-colored stain that was identified as mucus, presumably from the nose or mouth.[11]

JonBenét's right wrist was tied with a white cord.[11] Wrapped around her neck was a cord, similar to the one tied around her wrist, with one of the tail ends looped several times around a wooden stick.[11] A deep, horizontal furrow caused by the ligature encircled the entire neck, consistent with strangulation.[11] In addition, the skin above and below the furrow contained areas of abrasion and bleeding under the skin known as "petechial hemorrhage."[11]

Several areas with abrasions and/or petechial hemorrhage were also present on the face, near the chin, on both shoulders, and on the left lower back and left lower leg.[11] These burn-like marks, which were absent in photographs of JonBenét taken on Christmas morning, were later interpreted by some experts as consistent with having been caused by a stun gun, something the Ramsey family did not own and that was never found.[12]

It appeared JonBenét had been hit on the head. A skull fracture was clearly identified at the autopsy, as well as fresh hemorrhage and contusions in various areas of the brain.[13] There were no rib fractures.[13]

While both lungs and the heart were normal, there were occasional scattered petechial hemorrhages on the surfaces of each organ.[13] And as expected in such a young child, there was no evidence of atherosclerotic plaque in the aorta or in any of the cardiac arteries.[13] As for the remaining major organs—the spleen, adrenal gland, kidneys, liver, pancreas, stomach, gallbladder, and bowels—they were all normal and unremarkable.[13]

A small amount of dried blood was found on and around the vagina and inside the vaginal orifice.[13] An abrasion involving the hymen was also apparent.[13] Wood fragments from the paintbrush used to create the garrote with which JonBenét was strangled were found inside the vagina.[14] Yet, despite these genital abnormalities, Meyer did not provide an opinion whether JonBenét had been sexually assaulted, presumably because the findings were inconclusive.

Toxicology analysis did not detect any drugs or alcohol in JonBenét's blood.[15]

Cause and Manner of Death

In summarizing his final diagnosis, Meyer noted the autopsy findings related to strangulation, head injuries, and the various abrasions to the face, shoulders, legs, and vagina.[15] "The cause of death of this six year old female is asphyxia by strangulation associated with craniocerebral trauma," Meyer concluded.[15] The manner of death was a homicide.[15] I found nothing in the autopsy report to dispute Meyer's conclusions.

Life, Career, and the Police Investigation

JonBenét was born on August 6, 1990, in Atlanta, Georgia, but a year later, the Ramsey family moved to Colorado.[16] Patsy Ramsey had been Miss West Virginia in 1977, so it was only natural she would urge her daughter, who was a pretty, blond-haired girl with green eyes and a ready smile, to compete in child beauty pageants.[17]

Over the first six years of her life, JonBenét won at least eight beauty contests, including Little Miss Colorado.[18] On December 17, 1996, she was crowned Little Miss Christmas, after modelling in several outfits and performing "Rockin' Around the Christmas Tree."[18]

At the time JonBenét was murdered, the Boulder Police Department had very little experience conducting a murder investigation.[19] The lead investigator had never been involved in a homicide, and one of the detectives had no prior experience in solving a murder.[20] And while a new officer took over the case in October 1997, apparently he too had only limited homicide experience.[21] As a result, police made several mistakes in their investigation. They failed to secure the crime scene properly and did not interview the Ramsey parents and their son separately the day JonBenét's body was discovered.[21] In addition, information, some of which was confidential, was released without proper authorization, which may have undermined the investigation.[21]

Almost from the beginning, police focused their attention on John and Patsy Ramsey.[21] However, the Ramseys continued to claim their innocence, providing police with writing, hair and DNA samples, and even submitting to detailed interviews on April 30, 1997.[22]

The media speculated that JonBenét's brother may have been responsible for his sister's death. However, in May 1999, a spokeswoman for the Boulder County District Attorney's Office stated, "To this day, Burke Ramsey is not considered a suspect."[23]

One of the most crucial pieces of evidence in the murder investigation was the ransom note. It was three pages long, was addressed only to John Ramsey, and it was written with a fiber-tip pen on paper taken from the middle of a pad in the Ramsey residence.[23] Six handwriting experts, four hired by the police and two by the Ramseys, concluded that John Ramsey did not write the note.[23] The experts also agreed the likelihood Patsy Ramsey wrote the ransom note was very low.[23] At the same time, handwriting analysis did not eliminate other people who were under suspicion as possible authors of the note.[23]

In March 1997, the Boulder District Attorney's Office hired Andrew Louis Smit, a well-respected and highly experienced homicide investigator, to assist in the case.[23] After he reviewed all the evidence, Smit concluded that JonBenét was subdued by an intruder using a stun gun and was then taken from her bedroom to the basement, sexually assaulted, tortured, and murdered.[23] However, in September 1998, after the Boulder Police Department failed to investigate leads pointing to an intruder as the possible killer of JonBenét, Smit resigned.[23]

There was substantial evidence to support Smit's theory of an intruder as the person likely responsible for JonBenét's death.[23] Leaves and debris similar to those found inside a window well that covered three windows facing the back of the house and opening onto the playroom were found on the basement floor.[23] The same debris was also present in the wine cellar where JonBenét's body was found.[23] In addition, the suitcase found in the basement below the window well contained a pillow sham, a duvet, and a Dr. Seuss book, items the Ramseys owned but did not place in the suitacase.[23]

Police conducted several experiments and found that it was possible for a person to enter the basement of the Ramsey home through the center window in the window well.[23] Also, JonBenét had apparently told her friend's mother on December 25 that Santa Claus was going to pay her a "special" visit after Christmas and that it was a secret.[23] However, the person who may have said that to JonBenét has never been identified.[23]

Other evidence supporting the intruder theory included the way JonBenét's body was bound.[23] It suggested it was done by someone who had experience tying complicated knots and using a garrote.[23] In addition, animal hair that did not match anything in the

Ramsey home was found on JonBenét's hands and on the black tape covering her mouth.[23] Lastly, a baseball bat not owned by the Ramsey family was found outside the house.[23] It was covered with fibers consistent with fibers in the carpet present in the Ramsey basement.[23]

Perhaps the most damning evidence supporting the possibility of an intruder was the presence of unidentified male DNA under JonBenét's fingernails and on her underwear.[23] The DNA did not match DNA of any Ramsey family member or anyone associated with the Ramseys.[24] And while police were unable to establish to whom boot prints and a palm print found in the basement and wine cellar door, respectively, belonged or when they were made, they didn't belong to anyone in the Ramsey family.[25]

Sometime in the summer of 1998, a grand jury was convened to investigate the murder of JonBenét.[25] The jury was discharged in October 1999, however, for lack of sufficient evidence to bring charges "beyond a reasonable doubt" against anyone, including any member of the Ramsey family.[26]

Nine years later, a Bode Technology Group laboratory reported that, using a new and highly sophisticated "touch DNA" scraping methodology, they had recovered male DNA from two areas of long johns worn by JonBenét the day her body was discovered.[27] Further, the male

DNA profile from the long johns was the same as the male DNA profile previously obtained from JonBenét's underwear.[27] Neither profile belonged to John or Burke Ramsey.[27] Based on this new evidence, the Boulder District Attorney's Office concluded that the DNA found on JonBenét's long johns and underwear belonged to a male intruder and that the Ramsey family were no longer suspects in the case.[27]

Conclusion

JonBenét's murder will undoubtedly forever be a case study for how not to conduct a forensic homicide investigation. A botched crime scene and infighting among the Boulder Police Department and the Boulder District Attorney's Office hampered resolution of the case.[28] Some have claimed the Ramseys, one of Boulder's wealthiest families at the time, had been treated too lightly by police and prosecutors.[29] Others have suggested that leads pointing to an intruder as the perpetrator of the crime were not pursued aggressively enough.[29]

At least two people, a convicted pedophile and a school teacher arrested in Thailand, confessed to murdering JonBenét.[30] However, they were eliminated as suspects when their DNA did not match DNA obtained from clothing worn by JonBenét the day her body was discovered.[30] Other potential suspects were also cleared by DNA analysis.[31]

In 2010, the Boulder District Attorney's Office transferred the investigation back to the Boulder Police Department.[32] "Some cases never get solved, but some do," Mark Beckner, the Boulder police chief, said at the time.[33] "And you can't give up."[33] However, ten years later, JonBenét's murder remains unsolved.

It now appears police are relying almost exclusively on DNA analysis to identify the person responsible for JonBenét's death. Mary T. Lacy, the Boulder district attorney, wrote in a 2008 apology letter to the Ramsey family, "We hope that we will one day obtain a DNA match from the CODIS [Combined DNA Index System] data bank that will lead to further evidence and to the solution of this crime."[34] So far, this has not happened.

Since December 25, 1996, the day JonBenét was murdered, Burke has graduated from Purdue University, Patsy Ramsey has died from ovarian cancer, and John Ramsey has remarried. Also, many of the principals involved in the investigation have moved on. Beckner, the Boulder police chief who took over the case in 2010, has retired, Lacy, the former Boulder district attorney who eliminated the Ramsey family as suspects, has focused her attention on preventing childhood sexual abuse, and Smit, the police investigator who came out of retirement to assist the Boulder Police Department, has died.[35]

The murder of JonBenét is now a cold case. More than twenty years have passed since she was murdered, but to date, no one has been apprehended for the horrific crime. Many believe the killer will never be caught.[36] They may be right. Only time will tell.

CHAPTER 13

Anna Nicole Smith

Died February 8, 2007

ON SEPTEMBER 7, 2006, Anna Nicole Smith, an actress and celebrity personality, gave birth in the Bahamas to a baby girl, but the baby's father was not named.[1] Then, while visiting his new half sister in the hospital, Smith's twenty-year-old son died from a lethal combination of methadone, an opioid medication, escitalopram, an antidepressant, and tamsulosin, medicine prescribed for urinary retention.[2] Five months later, Smith went to Fort Lauderdale, Florida, to purchase a luxury yacht and to sail it back to the Bahamas.[3]

Smith came down with stomach flu and was too sick to leave her room at the Seminole Hard Rock Hotel and Casino.[3] Her temperature was reportedly as high as 105 degrees, but she refused to go to the hospital, wanting to avoid the media frenzy. Instead, Smith was placed in an ice bath that dropped her temperature down to ninety-seven and was treated with the antiviral medication, oseltamivir, and the antibiotic ciprofloxacin, as well as with chloral hydrate, a sedative-hypnotic drug prescribed to help her sleep.[4] The next day, Smith seemed fine, so later that afternoon, she was given another dose of chloral hydrate, after which she slept for about two hours. When she awoke, she watched television until about 11:00 p.m. and then took a third dose of the sedative.

The following morning, Smith ate breakfast, took a bath, and watched more television.[4] The last time anyone saw her alive was at ten o'clock that night, sitting on the living room couch and watching television.[4]

At about one o'clock the following afternoon, Smith was found unresponsive in bed by a family friend.[4] Her bodyguard's wife, a registered nurse, immediately began to administer CPR until paramedics arrived shortly before two.[4] They tried to revive Smith with cardiopulmonary resuscitation, but they were unsuccessful.[4] She was pronounced dead at Memorial Regional Hospital at 2:49 p.m.[4] She was thirty-nine years old.

The Autopsy

Smith's autopsy was performed about twenty hours after she died. It lasted nearly six hours.[5] Besides Dr. Joshua A. Perper, the chief medical examiner of the Broward County Medical Examiner Office in Fort Lauderdale, Florida, who conducted the autopsy, and Dr. Gertrude M. Juste, an associate medical examiner who assisted Perper, others in attendance included three members of the medical staff, a forensic technician, the chief toxicologist, two forensic photographers, the morgue supervisor, and three members of the Broward Sheriff's Office and Seminole Police Department.[5]

"The body is clad in a light green hospital gown, which is intact, dry and clean," Perper wrote in the autopsy report.[5] It had no noticeable trauma to the skin or evidence of blunt force, gunshot wound, or asphyxiation, which immediately ruled out homicide as a possible cause of death.[5] Evidence of recent contusions on both shoulders were consistent with reports that Smith fell in the bathroom the night before she died.[5]

In her final days, Smith had been suffering from stomach flu, so I was especially interested to review the autopsy findings related to the gastrointestinal system. Although an ounce of a bloody fluid was found in her stomach, something that is commonly seen in terminal shock, the stomach wasn't ulcerated, which meant that the blood didn't originate from bleeding ulcers.[6] However, the duodenum, an area immediately beyond the stomach and before the small bowel, was minimally inflamed, and a yellowish fluid with thick, cloudy, particulate matter was present in the small bowel beyond the duodenum.[7] In addition, the spleen had a slightly increased number of inflammatory cells, a biological response to a viral or bacterial infection.[7] Together, these findings suggested that in the days prior to her death, Smith had been suffering from viral gastroenteritis, an infection of the digestive system.[7]

As expected, each of Smith's breasts contained an implant.[7] Also, there was a telltale sign of a well-healed scar on her abdomen consistent with having previously given birth by Caesarian section.[7] However, no ribs, sternum, or spine fractures were identified.[8]

A detailed examination of Smith's buttocks was undertaken because Smith had complained of pain in that area before she died. The examination revealed small scars on each buttock.[9] Perhaps most striking were the large number of cysts, some containing turbid, yellowish fluid, and abscesses with creamy, yellow-green pus, as well as scarred and fibrotic tissue and recent hemorrhagic needle tracts on her buttocks.[10] Cultures of the abscesses confirmed that Smith's chronic and severe pain was caused by a bacterial infection.[11]

Of the remaining autopsy findings, none of which contributed to Smith's death, the most significant were a mildly enlarged liver, a thyroid gland that showed some mild abnormality indicative of Hashimoto thyroiditis, a condition in which the thyroid gland is unable to produce enough thyroid hormone, and lungs with right-sided pleural adhesions, a common finding in people who have experienced repeated episodes of lung inflammation. [12] The heart and cardiovascular system were normal, the lungs were of normal weight, the kidneys were unremarkable with no structural abnormalities, and the thymus was absent.[12]

At this point, it was easy to exclude pneumonia, a blood clot, heart disease, stroke, cancer, and internal bleeding as possible causes of Smith's death.[13] And while Smith had suffered from a bacterial infection in her buttocks prior to her death, sepsis was also excluded since bacteria were not identified in Smith's blood, urine, stool, or cerebrospinal fluid.[13] The question still remained, however, why did Smith die? As nearly always in such a situation, the answer would have to reveal itself in the toxicology report.

Cause and Manner of Death

The most significant substance found in Smith's blood was an extremely large amount of the potent sedative-hypnotic drug chloral hydrate.[14] This was consistent with reports Smith routinely took three to six times more chloral hydrate than she was prescribed and that she would sometimes drink the medication right out of the bottle.[14] Coincidentally, the same drug was also implicated in Marilyn Monroe's death, someone who Smith had idolized and who she had tried to emulate.[14] In addition, four different tranquilizers—diazepam, lorazepam, clonazepam, and oxazepam—were detected at low, therapeutic levels in Smith's blood, as well as the antihistamine diphenhydramine.[15] When taken together, these drugs, all with sedative properties, enhanced the sedative effect of chloral hydrate, causing extreme drowsiness, depressed respiration, changes in heart rate and heart rhythm, coma, and ultimately death from respiratory depression.

Several other drugs were identified in Smith's blood at therapeutic levels, but none had contributed to her death.[16] These included topiramate, a drug prescribed for weight reduction, ciprofloxacin, an antibiotic with which Smith had been treated at the Seminole Hard Rock Hotel, the over-the-counter pain reliever acetaminophen, and atropine, a drug used by emergency medical services first responders when they tried to restart Smith's heart.[16]

After I reviewed the relevant records, I agreed with Perper's conclusion that Smith died from drug intoxication caused by an overdose of chloral hydrate combined with low, therapeutic levels of five different prescription medications.[16] But was Smith's death an intentional attempt at suicide or an unfortunate accident?

Smith had developed many classic symptoms of clinical depression after the death of her son.[17] In addition, she had just given birth, a time when some women experience postpartum depression.[17] And while she was involved in four lawsuits that undoubtedly put additional strain on her already fragile mental state, her general mood in her final days appeared to be upbeat.[17] Thoughts of suicide would have been inconsistent with Smith's plans for furniture shopping and dancing lessons and a future in the Bahamas.[17]

Although Smith had a long history of prescription drug use and for self-medicating, she probably was unaware of the danger posed by polypharmacy, simultaneously taking six different drugs with sedative properties, all of which depressed the central nervous system.[18] After considering all of these factors, Perper concluded, and I agreed, that the most likely explanation for Smith's death was that it was an accident.[18]

Life and Career

Born in Houston, Texas, Smith spent a short time in Mexia, a city located forty miles east of Waco, after her parents divorced.[19] When she was only fourteen years old and in her junior year, Smith dropped out of high school. [20] "It's not like we're proud," Glenn McGuire, a math teacher at Mexia High School said when he heard of Smith's death.[21] "You don't see signs when you come into town saying 'This is the home of Anna Nicole Smith,'" the school's principal agreed.[21] "There are better things to be known for. It is not a path that I would recommend to our students."

After she left high school, Smith worked at minimum wage jobs, including one at a local restaurant where she met Billy Wayne Smith, a seventeen-year-old cook who she married in 1985.[22] Nine months later, she gave birth to a baby boy, but within a year, Smith and her husband separated and eventually divorced. Smith and her new baby moved back to Houston, where she took on odd jobs at Red Lobster and Wal-Mart.[22]

It was while in Houston that Smith saw a large neon sign of a woman dancing and thought, *I can dance*, not realizing that the place was a strip club where she would be expected to dance topless and do lap dances. [23] It was there she met the eighty-six-year-old oil mogul

J. Howard Marshall.[23] Married twice before and sixty years Smith's senior, Marshall was instantly smitten. He began to spend much time with Smith, lavishing her with expensive jewelry and paying more than $14,000 for her silicone implants.[24] "I was flat-chested growing up," Smith told Regis Filbin in a television interview. [25] "Everything I have is because of them," she said, pointing to her breasts.[26]

Smith and Marshall, now nearing ninety, were married in 1994 at the White Dove Wedding Chapel in Houston, three years after they met.[27] The bride had a creosote tan, a blond bouffant hairdo, and wore a confection of tulle; the groom, dapper in his white tux, arrived in a wheelchair.[28] After the ceremony, Smith gave her new husband a kiss and then was whisked off to the airport to fly to Europe for a modeling job.[28]

Sometime before she married Marshall, Smith submitted nude photos of herself to *Playboy* magazine. Surprisingly, Hugh Hefner, founder and editor in chief of *Playboy*, selected her for the cover of the March 1992 issue and for the 1993 Playmate of the Year.[29] It was just the break Smith had been looking for. Paul Marciano, one of the founders of Guess Jeans, saw Smith's photo in *Playboy* and decided to feature her as the new face of his brand.[30] "I changed her name," Marciano recalled in a 2017 interview.[30] She didn't know how beautiful she was, he said—six feet tall, bigger than life, with a magnetic personality, yet fragile and vulnerable.[30] Other modeling assignments soon followed, including for the Swedish clothing company H&M. Smith's photo appeared on billboards in Sweden and Norway and reportedly was responsible for having caused several car accidents.[31]

Smith began to appear in films, acting along with Leslie Nielsen in *Naked Gun 33 1/3,* with John Travolta in *Be Cool,* and in the science fiction comedy *Illegal Aliens.* Her performances in *To the Limit*, *Skyscraper* and in *Wasabi Tuna* drew poor reviews, and her appearances on several television shows such as *Sin City Spectacular*, *Anna Nicole Smith: Exposed, Veronica's Closet,* and *Ally McBeal* were less than stellar.[32] Then, despite the popularity of *The Anna Nicole Show*, the reality show was cancelled after two seasons.[33]

In 2004, Smith was a presenter at the American Music Awards.[34] Slurring her words, she seemed high and out of control.[34] Also in 2004, Smith was a presenter at the G-Phoria, a video game show awards ceremony, when her entire left breast popped out of her dress.[35] And at the 2005 MTV Australia Video Music Awards, Smith lowered the front of her dress all the way down to her waist, showing off her panties and breasts, her nipples barely covered with pasties of the Australia Video Music Awards logo.[36] "And the best music nominee video is …"

she said, but nobody listened.[36] Everybody wondered what outrageous thing Smith would do next.

Thirteen months after he married Smith, Marshall died from stomach cancer.[37] It was the beginning of Smith's nearly twenty-year-long legal battle for a share of her husband's fortune, allegedly worth more than $1.6 billion. [38] Although Smith wasn't named in the will, she claimed Marshall promised her half of his estate.[38] But in the end, a judge rejected all efforts by Smith's estate to secure $44 million in compensatory damages and to sanction the estate of her husband's son, E. Pierce Marshall, who died sometime during the litigation battle.[39]

Conclusion

Smith wasn't famous because of her acting. She wasn't even well known because of her extraordinary five-feet-eleven-inch height, her enormous silicone breasts and platinum-blonde hair, or even for being the 1993 *Playboy* Playmate of the Year and a former model for Guess Jeans and Lane Bryant.[40] What Smith was most famous for was for her second marriage to a nearly ninety-year-old billionaire oil tycoon when she was just twenty-six years old.[40] "He is the only person in my life who doesn't care what other people say about me," she said about her husband in an interview with Larry King.[40] "He truly loves me, and I love him for it."[40] Many people doubted Smith's sincerity, calling her a gold digger, but she didn't care. "It just so happens that I get turned on by liver spots," she quipped.[40]

After Smith died, many men came forward to claim they had sired her new daughter, but DNA analysis revealed it was Larry Birkhead, one of Smith's former boyfriends.[41]

"I want to be the new Marilyn Monroe and find my own Clark Gable," Smith had proclaimed in one of her interviews.[42] "There is no comparison," Richard Walter, a film producer, said when he heard of Smith's interest. [42] "Marilyn Monroe was an artist, a real performer, able to evoke in audiences a real empathy and a passion." The only similarity between Smith and Monroe was they both died young from an overdose of chloral hydrate.[42]

Like many young girls before her, Smith was a high school dropout who wanted to achieve fame and stardom. [42] "I want it so bad. I've tried so hard my whole life. I'm kind-hearted, and I give, give, give. I think maybe it's my time to receive," Smith said.[42] She pursued her dream with her huge, silicone breast implants, a marriage to an octogenarian, and outrageous behavior. "I've always liked attention," Smith said.[43] "I didn't get it very much growing up, and I always wanted to be, you know, noticed."

People ridiculed Smith, but she didn't pay them any mind. Many thought her life was "stranger than fiction" while others called her a "professional hot mess."[44] Still others called her behavior and antics "pathetic." [45] Birkhead disagreed. "The thing about Anna … it was almost like [she had] a split personality," he said.[46] "When the camera was going, she was a whole different thing … that was more, to me, an act than it was the real person, who she was."

In her final days, Smith was surrounded by an entourage of friends, acquaintances, and hangers-on, but none of them stopped her from overdosing on prescription medications. "Anna called the shots in Anna's life and everyone close to her knows that," said Lilly Ann Sanchez, an attorney.[47] "She was a very dear friend who meant a great deal to *Playboy* and to me personally," Hefner told reporters when he heard of Smith's passing.[48]

There was another side to Smith that wasn't well publicized. She was foremost a mother who loved her son very much. Like River Phoenix, she was also a supporter of People for the Ethical Treatment of Animals' campaign against the use of fur, certain pet foods, and cruelty to animals, as well as a supporter of gay and lesbian rights. [49] She even attended the thirty-fifth annual Los Angeles gay, lesbian, bisexual, and transgender Pride parade in 2005.[50]

Smith became a pop culture icon and a reality star before reality stars became popular.[51] Some may remember her as just another one of Hollywood's beautiful women who died much too young, but because of her little-known admirable personality traits, Smith would surely outrank many other reality celebrities.

CHAPTER 14

Heath Ledger
Died January 22, 2008

ON JANUARY 22, 2008, Heath Ledger's housekeeper arrived at his fourth-floor apartment in Manhattan's SoHo district in New York City at approximately twelve thirty in the afternoon.[1] When she went into the bathroom to change a lightbulb, she passed Ledger, an actor and a rising Hollywood film star. He was in bed, lying on his stomach, snoring, with a sheet pulled up around his shoulders.[1] About two hours later, Diana Wolozin came to give Ledger his regularly scheduled massage.[1] After knocking on his bedroom door and receiving no reply, Wolozin opened the door, only to find Ledger still in bed.[1] She set up her massage table and shook Ledger's shoulder, trying to wake him, but he didn't respond.[1] Realizing he was unconscious, she used Ledger's cell phone to call his friend in California, actress Mary-Kate Olsen, who offered to contact a private security service in New York to provide assistance.[1]

Wolozin called 911 at 3:26 p.m. and told the dispatcher that Ledger wasn't breathing.[1] Personnel from emergency medical services arrived within minutes. Responders from the security service that Olson had contacted showed up shortly thereafter.[1] CPR was performed and a cardiac defibrillator was used, but Ledger couldn't be resuscitated.[1] He was pronounced dead at 3:36 p.m.[1]

The Autopsy

In a statement released on February 6, 2008, a representative from the office of the chief medical examiner of the city of New York said, "Mr. Heath Ledger died as the result of acute intoxication by the combined effects of oxycodone, hydrocodone, diazepam, temazepam, alprazolam, and doxylamine."[2] Oxycodone and hydrocodone are opioid painkillers often prescribed in combination with aspirin or acetaminophen, respectively, diazepam, temazepam, and alprazolam are tranquilizers and antianxiety medications, and doxylamine is an antihistamine drug present in many over-the-counter sleep aids.

Since neither the toxicology report nor the autopsy report was available for review, I was unable to verify the levels of drugs found in Ledger's blood or whether Ledger had any anatomical abnormalities that would have contributed to his death. However, if one is to believe Ledger's father, "none of the medications was taken in excess of the prescribed dose."[3] Nevertheless, simultaneously taking two opioid drugs and three benzodiazepine tranquilizers, all of which are potent central nervous system and respiratory depressants, along with an antihistamine with sedative properties, can be lethal and is a typical example of how polypharmacy can cause severe respiratory depression and death.

Two months before he died, Ledger told a reporter he had difficulty falling asleep.[3] "Last week I probably slept an average of two hours a night," he said.[3] "I couldn't stop thinking. My body was exhausted, and my mind was still going."[3] The presence of six sedative drugs in his blood is consistent with Ledger's attempts to relieve his insomnia.[3]

Cause and Manner of Death

Police determined that foul play was not involved in Ledger's death.[3] However, they were unable to establish how Ledger obtained the various drugs that were detected in his blood.[3] The coroner ruled the cause of Ledger's death as drug intoxication and the manner of death an accident.[4]

Life and Career

Born in 1979 in Australia's western city of Perth, Ledger's first role in a feature film was in the 1997 low-budget, Australian movie *Blackrock*.[5] *Two Hands*, a crime thriller, and the teen comedy *10 Things I Hate About You* followed two years later.[6] However, afraid he would be typecast as a teen heartthrob, Ledger turned down offers for similar parts and instead accepted supporting roles in the war drama *The Patriot,* a 2000 Mel Gibson film, and as a prison guard in *Monster's Ball* (2001).[7] By 2005, Ledger had been featured in leading roles in at least four films.[8] "For me, acting is more about self-exploration," Ledger said in one interview.[9] "I've learned a lot about myself in order to learn about the craft."[9]

Ledger's groundbreaking performance was as a gay cowboy in *Brokeback Mountain*, but it wasn't the first time he portrayed a gay man. Nine years earlier, he appeared as a gay cyclist in *Sweat*, an Australian television series about Olympic hopefuls in a school for athletically gifted students.[9] The show was cancelled after twenty-six episodes, but it gave Ledger the understanding he needed to play Ennis Del Mar in *Brokeback Mountain*. He was awarded an Oscar for Best Actor for his performance in that role. He was only twenty-six years old.

After *Brokeback Mountain*, Ledger played the Joker in the 2008 film *The Dark Knight*.[9] "'The Joker,' so far, is definitely the most fun I've had with any character," he said at the time.[9] "He's just out of control—no empathy, he's a sociopath, a psychotic, mass-murdering clown."[9] Unfortunately, he didn't get to see the film released.

Unlike Marlon Brando, to whom he was often compared, Ledger never took acting lessons or studied method acting at the Actors' Studio in New York City.[9] "At the end of the day, it all comes down to my instincts," he said.[9] Brian Helgeland, director of *A Knight's Tale,* compared Ledger to another famous actor. "When Heath smiles, it's Errol Flynn."[10]

Some of his fans feared Ledger became addicted to sleeping pills because of his all-consuming obsession with his characters, especially the Joker. They thought that's what led to his death, but there's no evidence to support this theory.[11] Although Ledger died from a combination of six different sedatives, he had been taking sleeping pills ever since he was a teenager.[11]

When he heard that Ledger died, Gibson, who played Ledger's father in *The Patriot*, said, "I had such great hope for him. He was just taking off and to lose his life at such a young age is a tragic loss."[12] Eric Roberts, who worked with Ledger in *The Dark Knight*, agreed. "He was a wonderful guy, he was a wonderful actor, he had a wonderful future ahead of him."[12]

Ledger was very curious about acting and art, in general, and this was readily apparent in the documentary film *I Am Ledger*.[13] Always with a camera, whether Polaroid, still, or movie, Ledger filmed the mundane as well as his own reflection, leaving behind numerous recordings that were incorporated into the documentary about his short life. One reviewer wrote, Ledger was "an ever curious, hyperactive young man who was living on borrowed time."[13]

It is tempting to speculate what might have been had Ledger lived, but it would be an exercise in futility. Extremely talented with an on-screen charisma, Ledger was serious about his craft. "It all comes down to being willing to be taught," he said in a *Vanity Fair* interview on the set of *The Patriot*.[14] "The day I stop having fun, I'll just walk away."[14] Unfortunately, he never got a chance to see that day.

Conclusion

In the United States, more than 30 percent of overdoses involve a combination of opioids and benzodiazepines. [15] According to the National Institute on Drug Abuse, or NIDA, "combining opioids and benzodiazepines can be unsafe because both types of drugs sedate and suppress breathing—the cause of overdose fatality—in addition to impairing cognitive functions."[15] In one study, the overdose death rate among patients who received a combination of these central nervous system depressant drugs was ten times higher than among those who received opioids alone.[16] To highlight the dangers posed by prescribing opioids and benzodiazepines together, the Food and Drug Administration, or FDA, requires a black box warning on the label of each drug.[17]

"Heath's accidental death [should serve] as a caution to the hidden dangers of combining prescription medications, even at low dosage," Ledger's father said in his statement after his son's death.[18] It was a warning that was appropriate in 2008, the year Ledger died, and is even more fitting today.

CHAPTER 15

Michael Jackson

Died June 25, 2009

THE FINAL REHEARSAL for Michael Jackson's fifty sold-out concerts at London's O2 arena was held on the evening of Wednesday June 24, 2009.[1] Jackson, a multitalented musical entertainer, was in good physical shape, upbeat and very energetic, and was especially excited about the opening number in which an illuminated sphere floated away from him out into the audience and then returned, landing in his hand before burning in a blaze of light.[2] "He was grinning from ear to ear," Dorian Holley, Jackson's longtime vocal director, said of the rehearsal.[2]

Sometime after midnight, Jackson returned from the Staples Center in downtown Los Angeles, where the rehearsal was held, to his rented eight-bedroom house in Holmby Hills.[2] Dr. Conrad R. Murray, Jackson's personal physician, was already there.[2] Murray had been treating Jackson's chronic insomnia with powerful sedative drugs, so it wasn't unusual to see his car parked in the driveway.[2]

Jackson had been singing and dancing for three hours. His heart was racing, and his elevated blood sugar and adrenaline levels were undoubtedly keeping him alert and his brain active. Unwilling to give his body time to unwind naturally, he immediately began to complain to Murray that he wanted a sedative to help him sleep.

To calm Jackson down, Murray gave him an oral dose of diazepam, a tranquilizer, at about one thirty in the morning, but the drug had no appreciable effect.[2] A half hour later, he gave Jackson a different sedative, lorazepam.[2] For more rapid absorption, he administered the drug directly into Jackson's vein, but Jackson remained awake.[2] Over the next five and a half hours, Murray gave Jackson three doses of two different benzodiazepine tranquilizers, midazolam and lorazepam, but he still wouldn't fall asleep. Then, at 10:40 a.m., Murray relented to Jackson's demands and administered propofol, a potent general anesthetic he had given him in the past.[2] Phone logs would later reveal that after Murray administered the propofol, he left Jackson alone for half an hour. When he returned, Jackson wasn't breathing.[2] Murray and Jackson's bodyguard immediately began to administer CPR, but by the time paramedics arrived, Jackson had no pulse.[2] He was transported to the Ronald Reagan UCLA Medical Center where, despite heroic measures, he was pronounced dead.[2] He was fifty years old.

The Autopsy

Dr. Rogers looked at the body as it lay on the gurney in the autopsy room. Although he had already conducted the autopsy of several famous people during his tenure with the medical examiner-coroner's office of the county of Los Angeles, this one was different. The African American man on the gurney was a popular singer and entertainer whose music he had enjoyed countless of times. "The body is identified by toe tags and is that of an unembalmed refrigerated adult black male," Rogers wrote in his report.[3]

Jackson's scalp had no fractures, but the head, which was covered with a wig, was balding in the front.[3] The body had many scars, including a two-inch surgical scar in the lower abdomen, as well as several tattoos.[3] The skin had patches of light and dark pigmented areas, a condition known as vitiligo, for which Jackson had been treated with monobenzone and hydroquinone cream until he died. As for the mouth, it had evidence of dental implants, root canal, and metallic dental caps.[3]

What struck me the most as I reviewed the autopsy report was the excellent physical shape Jackson was in prior to his death.[3] The cardiovascular system had no evidence of plaque, the heart size and weight were in the normal range, and the heart muscle, heart chambers, and heart valves were not defective.[3] All in all, Jackson had a low risk for a heart-related event.[3] And while the brain had some mild vascular congestion and mild calcification, it wasn't an unusual finding in men of Jackson's age.[3]

Other autopsy findings, none of which contributed to Jackson's death, included three slightly raised nodules on the left side of the larynx consistent with tonsillar tissue, three relatively firm masses in the left lower lung lobe, and lungs that were moderately congested and inflamed, which may have caused Jackson some difficulty breathing.[4]

A small mass located near Jackson's left adrenal gland was normal when viewed under a microscope.[5] Also, a small polyp in his colon was later identified as a benign tubular adenoma.[5] Had Jackson lived, the polyp could have been easily removed during a routine colonoscopy.[6]

Like many men in his age group, Jackson had a moderately enlarged nodular prostate that, although not cancerous, caused him to urinate more frequently than normal.[7] This explained why tamsulosin, a drug often prescribed to reduce the urgent need to urinate in men suffering from an enlarged prostate, also known as benign prostatic hypertrophy, was found in Jackson's room.[7] Furthermore, Jackson had mild to moderate degenerative osteoarthritis in the joints of several of his fingers, minimal degeneration of the lower spine, and mild atherosclerotic plaque in the arteries of both legs.[7] These findings undoubtedly were an occupational hazard caused by his long-term strenuous and unique style of dancing.

Cause and Manner of Death

My review of the autopsy report failed to reveal any anatomical changes that would explain why Jackson died. But when I reviewed the toxicology report, I noted the presence of several drugs in Jackson's blood, all of which had been administered by Murray. These included an excessive amount of propofol, a large amount of the tranquilizer lorazepam, as well as low levels of lidocaine, a local anesthetic, and the sedative midazolam.[7] This was the smoking gun that led me to the indisputable conclusion that Jackson died from respiratory and cardiovascular collapse caused by acute propofol intoxication accentuated by a large amount of lorazepam, with therapeutic amounts of lidocaine and midazolam as contributing factors in his death.[7]

Rogers concluded that Jackson's death was caused by acute propofol intoxication with benzodiazepine as a contributing factor.[7] He labeled the manner of death a homicide since Murray breached the standard of care when he administered the drugs in a nonhospital setting, in the absence of an appropriate medical indication, and without the recommended equipment for patient monitoring, precision dosing, and resuscitation.[7]

Found guilty of involuntary manslaughter, Murray served two of the four years to which he was sentenced in prison.[8] At his trial, his defense attorney suggested that Jackson had self-administered more propofol when Murray was out of the room, but the jury wasn't convinced.[8] It would have been extremely difficult for Jackson to do so, considering the catheter was in his left leg and the injection port was thirteen and a half centimeters away from the tip of the catheter.[9] He would have had to bend his knee or sit up in a very awkward position to reach the injection port and to push the barrel of the syringe.[9]

Life and Career

Jackson was the eighth of ten children of Katherine and Joseph Jackson.[10] His mother enjoyed singing, often leading her children in singalongs and teaching them to harmonize, whereas his father played guitar in a band called the Falcons.[11]

When Jackson's father saw that his three oldest sons were interested in music, he bought them a guitar and a bass and began to groom them into a musical group called the Jackson Brothers.[11] But in 1964, when Jackson was only six years old, he joined the group as its lead vocalist, and later, when his brother Marlon was added, the group became known as the Jacksons.[12]

The Jackson 5 built a strong local following and was booked into black nightclubs in Chicago and Gary, Illinois. Later, they toured black venues in the United States, where they opened for the Temptations, Jackie Wilson, Etta James, and James Brown.[13] In 1967, the group won Amateur Night at the Apollo Theater in New York.[13]

Berry Gordy, founder of Motown Records, signed the Jackson 5 to his record label in 1968.[14] Their first album, *Diana Ross Presents the Jackson 5*, hit the music charts in December of the following year. Their song "I Want You Back" reached number one on the Billboard Hot 100 chart shortly thereafter, with other chart-topping songs soon following.[15] But despite their overwhelming success, conflicts over creative control led the group to leave Motown Records and to sign with Epic Records under their new name, the Jacksons, with Randy Jackson replacing his brother Jermaine, who had married Berry Gordy's daughter and chose to remain at Motown Records to begin a solo career.[16]

Jackson was also interested in a solo career. After he signed with Epic Records, he began to work on his own album with Quincy Jones, the well-respected composer, arranger, and music director.[17] *Off the Wall* contained the Grammy Award–winning single "Don't Stop 'Till You Get Enough."[18] His next album, *Thriller*, was released in 1982. It included seven Top 10 hits and won eight Grammys, including Album of the Year, and eight American Music Awards.[19] The album became the best-selling album in history, with more than 110 million copies sold worldwide.[20] Two other highly successful albums, *Bad* and *Dangerous*, established Jackson as the "King of Pop," a term Elizabeth Taylor, the actress, bestowed upon Jackson when she presented him with the 1989 Soul Train Heritage Award.[21]

Motown Records' twenty-fifth anniversary celebration had already been held at the Pasadena Civic Auditorium in Pasadena, California, two months earlier, but NBC taped the event and had decided to air it on May 16, 1983.[22] The program began on a sluggish note, with dance numbers by the Lester Wilson Dancers.[23] But sometime in the middle of the program, the Jackson 5 was introduced to sing "I Want You Back," "The Love You Save," and "Never Can Say Goodbye."[23] When the group completed its routine, Jackson, one of the five brothers, remained on the stage. He was dressed in a black jacket with sequins that twinkled every time the lights hit it at just the right angle, a silver lamé shirt, black slacks with high cuffs, white socks that glittered, and loafers, and on his left hand, he wore a white glove with twelve hundred rhinestones.[24] Staring at the audience, Jackson smiled his infectious smile.[25]

"Thank you. Oh, you're beautiful. Thank you. Thank you," Jackson said and waited for the audience to settle down. "Those were good songs. I like those songs a lot, but especially"—he stopped for a dramatic pause and then added—"I like"—pausing again—"the new songs." [25] In one quick motion, he turned, reached down for his black fedora, bent his knees, and, grabbing his crotch, began to thrust his pelvis in several forward motions as the familiar beat of his latest song, "Billie Jean," from his highly successful, recently released album, *Thriller*, began to play.[26] Everyone in the audience went wild with raw, unbridled animal excitement.

Jackson lip-synched to the original soundtrack, his body in constant motion, kicking his feet up to a perfect horizontal, tapping his toes to the beat, spinning many revolutions, and raising his fists to his face.[27] He had the audience in the palm of his white-gloved, shimmering hand, and there was no stopping him. And then, at exactly 3:35 minutes into the song, the unimaginable happened. Jackson appeared to walk on air as he sang, "She said I am the one," while seemingly gliding backward. The audience screamed.

The moonwalk took no more than two seconds, but it was magical and beyond belief.[28] And just for good measure, Jackson repeated the move at 4:32 minutes into the song, about fifteen seconds before he finished his performance and then left the stage. A new era in musical entertainment had begun, resembling the second coming of the Beatles.

Jackson became famous not only for his singing but also for his extraordinarily astonishing dance moves. But he wasn't the first to do so. Long before he introduced the moonwalk, there was Elvis Presley, who sexually gyrated his hips as he sang to swooning and adoring fans.[29] But when Jackson introduced the "antigravity lean," a move that involved achieving a forty-five degree lean while keeping the spine straight, it seemed beyond the capability of any man.[30] The secret was in a specially patented shoe with a triangular slot near the heel. When it engaged a metallic peg that emerged from the stage floor, it provided Jackson the extra support he needed to lean forward without falling over.[30] The illusion was incredible.

Conclusion

As an entertainer, Jackson could best be described as a modern-day Sammy Davis Jr. Like Jackson, Davis was an African American who began his entertainment career at a very young age, just three years old.[31] He first performed with his father and uncle as part of the Will Mastin Trio. But just like Jackson, Davis soon became the star of the group.[31] Davis was an extraordinary dancer and singer, just like Jackson, who eventually became an entertainment phenomenon in his own right.[31] However, unlike Jackson, Davis drew criticism from the black community for his support of President Richard Nixon during the Vietnam War and was confronted by strong prejudice and racism.[31] Nevertheless, that Jackson and Davis could be favorably compared is a testament to their talent and the love of their fans.

It is undeniable that Jackson was an entertainment sensation, the likes of which we may never see again. His career spanned more than forty-five years and reached dizzying heights when *Thriller* was released. But Jackson's career also plunged to the lowest of lows when allegations of child molestation began to surface before he died and continued to emerge even after his death. His legacy was forever tarnished, especially after the documentary *Leaving Neverland* was released in 2019.[32] It was this dichotomy that left fans unsure how to admire Jackson the entertainer while at the same time vilify Jackson, the man, for his alleged deviant behavior against children.

In show business, what you see may not always be what you get. It should be no surprise, then, that despite allegations of child molestation, the public continued to idolize Jackson because, in its collective mind, the entertainer was different from the man, and more importantly, the allegations had never been proven.

I choose to leave the question of how to reconcile the two sides of Michael Jackson to psychiatrists and psychologists. Any new revelations and accusations should be left to law enforcement authorities and medical professionals to evaluate and not to the popular press or the digital media. Instead, I think it's best to concentrate on the Jackson who entertained audiences for nearly half a century. But whatever the outcome of such future deliberations, one thing cannot be disputed. Jackson left an indelible mark on the consciousness of his audience, and his legacy as an entertainer will be forever remembered.

CHAPTER 16

Brittany Murphy

Died December 20, 2009

BRITTANY MURPHY, A young, talented actress, had been complaining of flu-like symptoms, shortness of breath, and abdominal pain in early December 2009.[1] She had had a history of diabetes, for which she had once been hospitalized, as well as a history of mitral valve prolapse, a condition in which the valve between the left ventricle and left atrium chambers of the heart does not close properly.[1] Either one of these problems potentially could have been the cause of her shortness of breath. As for her abdominal pain, it could have been related to her heavy menstrual bleeding.[1]

On December 20, still complaining of severe abdominal pain, Murphy went into the bathroom.[1] When she didn't come out thirty minutes later, her family opened the door and found Murphy lying unresponsive on the bathroom floor.[1] Paramedics were called, and when they arrived, they found Murphy pale and sweating, her pupils fixed and dilated.[1] She had no vital signs, and her blood sugar level was abnormally low. In full cardiac arrest, Murphy was immediately rushed by ambulance to Cedars-Sinai Medical Center in Los Angeles.

Blood tests revealed that Murphy's hemoglobin level, the iron-containing oxygen-transporting protein in red blood cells, was severely low.[1] Doctors diagnosed her with "hypochromatic, microcytic anemia," the most common form of which was iron-deficiency anemia.[1] Despite all attempts to resuscitate, Murphy was pronounced dead two hours after she arrived at the hospital.[1] She was thirty-two years old.

The Autopsy

Murphy's autopsy was conducted by Dr. Lisa A. Scheinin, a deputy medical examiner of the county of Los Angeles.[1] Scheinin had graduated from the University of Maryland School of Medicine with a specialty in forensic pathology.[2] "The body appears well-developed, normally muscular and slim, but not excessively thin," she wrote in the autopsy report.[3] There were no tattoos, surgical scars, or needle track marks.[3] The absence of rib or skeletal fractures or other traumatic injury supported police claim that foul play wasn't involved in Murphy's death. [3] As for the cardiovascular system, it appeared normal with no evidence of atherosclerotic plaque, narrowing of the coronary arteries or blood clots.

With the exception of the lungs, the lymphatic system, and the moderate distention of the small bowel, all of Murphy's major organs were normal.[3] The liver was smooth with a normal consistency, the stomach wasn't distended, both kidneys were normally situated, the urinary bladder was unremarkable, the thyroid and pituitary glands were as expected, and the urine was negative for glucose.[3] But while there was "moderate cerebral edema," fluid on the brain that was not an uncommon finding at autopsy, there was no evidence of hemorrhage beneath the scalp, which indicated Murphy didn't die from a concussion, as from a fall.[3]

The elevated infiltration of neutrophils and eosinophils in Murphy's small bowel, colon, and elsewhere was the first sign she may have been suffering from an infection before she died.[3] These specialized, disease-fighting white blood cells increase in number in response to a bacterial or viral infection, as well as in cancer. Errol Flynn's autopsy had a similar finding, a result of his several bouts of malaria. The presence of enlarged lymph nodes all over Murphy's body was consistent with the diagnosis of "generalized, but moderate lymphadenopathy," a disease of the lymph nodes.[3]

Both of Murphy's lungs had a "meaty consistency" and were heavy, dense, and filled with fluid, which accounted for the diagnosis of adult respiratory distress syndrome.[3] Dr. Koss, a pulmonologist and nephrologist, found evidence of moderate to severe pneumonia when he examined tissues of both lungs under a microscope.[3] Blood cultures identified Oxacillin-resistant Staphylococcus aureus bacteria, the most likely causative organism of the pneumonia.[3]

Murphy's iron blood level was at least 50 percent lower than normal, and her hematocrit, the proportion, by volume, of blood consisting of red blood cells, was also extremely low.[3] Both of these findings as well as Murphy's generalized pallor or paleness were consistent with her hospital diagnosis.[3] In addition, iron staining of the bone marrow, the gold standard for identifying chronic iron deficiency anemia, showed no evidence of iron deposits.[3] In the absence of gastrointestinal bleeding or trauma, the most likely explanation for Murphy's anemia was her history of heavy menstrual bleeding.

[3] In her weakened condition, she would have also been vulnerable to infection.

Cause and Manner of Death

Interestingly, Murphy was prescribed fourteen tablets of the antibiotic clarithromycin on November 16, about two weeks before she died.[3] However, she apparently didn't take any of them though because a full vial of the medication was found in her home.[3] Instead, she had been self-medicating with Vicodin, a pain medication consisting of the opioid hydrocodone and the nonnarcotic pain reliever acetaminophen, as well as with over-the-counter cold preparations containing the antihistamine chlorpheniramine, and with L-methamphetamine–containing nasal decongestants.[3] All of these drugs, as well as fluoxetine, a drug prescribed for depression, panic attacks, and an eating disorder, and chloridazepoxide, a medication taken for anxiety, were detected in Murphy's blood.[3]

I found no reason to dispute Scheinin's conclusions that Murphy's death from acquired community pneumonia was an accident.[3] Iron-deficiency anemia contributed to her weakened condition and, along with multiple drug intoxication, was a factor in her death.[3]

Life and Career

Murphy was only two years old when her parents divorced.
[3] Her father, who had been described as a member of the
Italian Mafia and one of the first to be prosecuted for
racketeering, was in and out of prison most of his life.
[4] As for her mother, "I think to call my mom and I best
friends is almost an insult to our relationship … She's the
greatest in the whole wide world, and I don't feel closer
to anyone," Murphy once said.[4]

Murphy became interested in performing at a very
young age. She began with dancing and voice lessons
when she was five years old, and by the time she was
twelve, she appeared on television commercials and
in sitcoms, such as *Murphy Brown* and *Blossom*.[4] In
1995, eighteen-year-old Murphy made her film debut
in *Clueless*.[4] She followed her performance with acting
roles in *Girl, Interrupted* (1999), *8 Mile* (2002), and *Sin
City* (2005).[4]

Sometime around November 2009, after filming
a scene in *The Caller* in Puerto Rico, Murphy was
unexpectedly dropped from the film because of her
alleged "poor attitude and spotty attendance."[4] It was a
devastating blow to an otherwise promising career.

When Murphy died, her family found it difficult to
accept Scheinin's conclusions, especially after Murphy's

husband died from the same ailments five months later.[5] Many people speculated that the two deaths were related and were caused by mold in the family home.[5] However, Ed Winter, the assistant chief coroner, disagreed.[5] Mold was specifically looked for as a causative agent in both autopsies, he said, but none was found.[6]

When a lab test found heavy metals in Murphy's hair, her father claimed Murphy had been poisoned.[7] "It was not at the level that would warrant reopening the case," Winter said, noting Murphy dyed her hair, and heavy metals are known to be present in people with dyed hair. [7] A rumor was then circulated that United States federal agents may have been responsible for the two deaths.[8] Both Murphy and her husband believed they were being watched after Murphy testified in a case on behalf of a Homeland Security employee. However, there was no evidence to support this claim either.

Conclusion

Murphy's death highlights the importance of seeking medical attention at the first sign of disease. "I had no idea she had pneumonia," Murphy's husband said at the time.[9] "I took very good care of my wife. She was on antibiotic and she was taking cough medicine and doing all the right things."[9] However, while Murphy was prescribed clarithromycin shortly before she died, she apparently didn't take the antibiotic.[10]

"I think that if [Murphy] had gotten medical attention instead of just delaying it, that they'd taken her to a doctor, she'd probably still be alive as we speak today," Winter told a reporter from *US Weekly*.[11] I can certainly agree. A new antibiotic might have been prescribed, or she might have been admitted to a hospital. As for Murphy's abnormally low iron and sugar levels, they too would have been corrected. It can almost be assured that the outcome would have probably been different had Murphy been seen by a physician as her respiratory symptoms worsened. Who knows? She might have entertained the public for several more years.

CHAPTER 17
Amy Winehouse
Died July 23, 2011

AMY WINEHOUSE, THE five-time Grammy Award–winning British singer-songwriter with a beehive hairdo, heavy eyeliner, and tattoos all over her body had a long history of alcohol and drug abuse that included heroin, cocaine, and marijuana, but she stopped using drugs shortly before she went on a trip to St Lucia.[1] Instead, she fell into on-again-off-again periods of alcohol consumption. She refused to see a psychiatrist to help battle her alcohol addiction and her eating disorder, fearing the psychiatric treatments could stifle her creativity.[1] Unwilling to tackle her addiction,

Winehouse was being treated with chlordiazepoxide to help her cope with symptoms of alcohol withdrawal.[1]

On Friday July 22, 2011, the day before her body was discovered in her apartment in North London, Winehouse visited her physician, Dr. Christina Romete. [1] "She was genuinely unwilling to follow the advice of doctors, being someone who wanted to do things her own way," Romete said in a written statement at Winehouse's inquest.[2] "She specifically said she did not want to die."[3] Andrew Morris, Winehouse's bodyguard, testified that he and Winehouse had watched YouTube videos of some of her performances that Friday evening, and he could hear her "laughing, listening to music, and watching TV" later that night.[3] According to Morris, the last time he spoke to Winehouse was at two o'clock on Saturday morning.[3] But when he checked on her at ten, he thought she was asleep, so he waited until two thirty or three o'clock in the afternoon before he entered her room again.[3] "She was in the same position as in the morning," he said at the inquest. "I checked her pulse, but I couldn't find one."[3]

When paramedics arrived, Winehouse was lying fully clothed on the bed.[3] Next to her was a laptop, and on the floor, beside the bed, were two large, empty vodka bottles. [3] Morris, who was the last person to see Winehouse alive, was shaken when paramedics confirmed that Winehouse was dead.[3] "She was like a sister to me," he said.[3]

The Autopsy

When the public first learned of Winehouse's death, people immediately assumed she died from a drug overdose. It was a logical conclusion, considering Winehouse had been abusing illicit drugs for many years. Since she died in England, Winehouse's death was investigated under the terms of Section 20 of the 1988 Coroner's Act, which states that a postmortem may be ordered when the coroner believes "there is reasonable cause to suspect that a person has died a violent or unnatural death or in any other way which would require an inquest."[4]

Police determined that Winehouse's death was not suspicious, but Suzanne Greenaway, the assistant deputy coroner, nevertheless opened a formal inquest and had a postmortem examination done on the body.[4]

Winehouse's autopsy report was not made public, so I wasn't able to review its findings. However, based on public records, it appears that no sign of injury was identified, nor were pill remnants found in Winehouse's stomach.[5] While toxicology analysis of Winehouse's blood did not detect any illicit drugs, alcohol was identified at more than five times the legal limit for drivers in England and in the United States.[6]

Cause and Manner of Death

The ability of the liver to metabolize alcohol was completely overwhelmed at Winehouse's level of intoxication. The alcohol poisoning severely depressed her central nervous system, slowed her heart rate, decreased her body temperature, sedated her to the verge of coma, and stopped her breathing. She died from respiratory depression.[7]

"She made tremendous efforts over the years" to quit drinking, Romete told authorities.[8] "I [warned] Amy over a long period of time ... about all the effects alcohol can have on the system, including heart problems, fertility problems, liver problems, respiratory depression, and death."[8]

At the October 26, 2011, inquest, Greenaway labeled the cause of Winehouse's death as "death by misadventure," an accidental death from alcohol poisoning.[9] "The unintended consequence of such potentially fatal levels [of alcohol]," Greenaway said, "was [Winehouse's] sudden and unexpected death."[9]

With the cause of Winehouse's death officially determined, her body was cremated and her ashes were laid to rest in a Jewish cemetery in London.[9] However, it was soon discovered Greenaway had not met the statutory requirement of having had at least five years of legal experience in Britain when she was appointed assistant deputy coroner by the North London coroner Dr. Andrew Scott Reid, who happened to have been her husband.[9] One month after the inquest, Greenaway resigned, and her husband resigned his post a year later.[10]

The conclusion of the inquest stymied, the verdict was thrown out, and a second inquest into Winehouse's death was undertaken on January 8, 2013.[11] At the second hearing, Dr. Shirley Radcliffe, the new interim coroner, announced that Winehouse died from alcohol intoxication, and the level of alcohol in her blood was "commonly associated with fatality."[11] The new verdict, "death by misadventure," was the same as the one of the earlier investigation, and it was now officially recorded.[12]

Life and Career

Winehouse was born in London.[13] A rebellious teenager, she pierced her nose, tattooed her body, and was expelled from school.[13] When she was thirteen years old, she taught herself to play the guitar.[13] At sixteen, she began to perform at clubs and to record demos.[13]

In 2003, Winehouse's debut album *Frank*, a mixture of jazz, pop, soul, and hip-hop, was nominated for several British music awards.[14] By then, Winehouse had already developed a strong liking for hard liquor and had often appeared at clubs too drunk to sing a whole set.[15] It was during this time that her boyfriend, Blake Fielder-Civil, whom Winehouse later married, allegedly introduced her to illicit drugs.[16]

By 2006, Winehouse's management company suggested that she enter rehab for alcohol and substance abuse, but she refused.[16] Instead, she dropped the company and wrote the song "Rehab" about her experience.[16] "Rehab" became the lead single for Winehouse's second album, *Back to Black*, reaching number nine on the pop charts in the United States.[16] *Back to Black* earned several British awards in 2007, including Best British Album.[16]

Drug use and strange behavior were now an integral part of Winehouse's life. In August 2007, she was hospitalized for overdosing on several drugs, including heroin, cocaine, Ecstasy, the anesthetic ketamine, and alcohol.[16] In October of the same year, Winehouse was arrested in Norway for possession of marijuana.[16] By mid-November, she showed up at one of her concerts so intoxicated she was booed off the stage.[16] Many in the audience walked out in midconcert.[16] And in January

2008, a video surfaced that showed Winehouse smoking crack cocaine.[16]

Winehouse was scheduled to perform live at the 2008 Grammy Awards, where she won several Grammys including for Best New Artist, Record of the Year, and Song of the Year. However, because of her "use and abuse of narcotics," she was denied a visa to enter the United States and had to perform by satellite.[16] Yet despite her success with *Back to Black* and being listed in the 2009 Guinness Book of World Records for "Most Grammy Awards Won by a British Female Act," Winehouse's addiction to drugs and alcohol was so debilitating that by 2011, at the young age of twenty-seven, she was dead.[16]

Conclusion

In death, Winehouse, like Jimi Hendrix and Janis Joplin before her, joined the ranks of the Twenty-Seven Club—a group of notable musicians who died at the age of twenty-seven.[17]

CHAPTER 18

Whitney Houston

Died February 11, 2012

FOUR DAYS BEFORE the fifty-fourth Annual Grammy Awards, Whitney Houston, an accomplished singer and actress, checked into the Beverly Hilton Hotel under the pseudonym Elizabeth Collins.[1] The Grammys was scheduled for Sunday at the Staples Center in Los Angeles, but the night before the event, Clive Davis planned to host his annual pre-Grammy party at the same hotel where Houston was staying.[2] "She was so looking forward to tonight even though she wasn't scheduled to perform," Clive Davis later *Rolling Stone* magazine.[2]

At about two thirty or three o'clock in the afternoon of Clive Davis's party, Mary Jones, Houston's personal assistant, laid out the gown that Houston was to wear that night and then went to pick up a package at Neiman Marcus, an exclusive department store.[3] "Take a bath and get ready for tonight," she told Houston on her way out.[3] But when Jones returned, she found Houston in the bathroom, lying facedown in the bathtub.[3] Jones immediately called the front desk and had them call 911. She then got Houston's personal bodyguard to help her pull Houston out of the tub.[3]

Paramedics arrived and placed Houston's nude body on the living room floor.[3] CPR was performed, as were other lifesaving measures, but Houston couldn't be resuscitated.[3] She was pronounced dead at 3:55 p.m.[3]

When police arrived, Houston's hotel suite was a study in contrasts. The living room appeared as if it was ready for a party with plates of food on three tables and an open bottle of champagne in an ice bucket, on top of a minibar.[3] However, next to the food were loose, unidentified tablets and capsules, as well as several prescription vials, a bottle of ibuprofen, and a number of blister packs of Midol, guaifenesin, a cold medication, and some tablets of the antihistamine diphenhydramine.[3] In the bedroom were more loose tablets and prescription bottles on top of a dresser and on top of a nearby table, as well as a bottle of a dietary supplement.[3]

In the bathroom, a small spoon with a white crystal-like substance was found on the counter, as well as a rolled up piece of white paper, a prescription bottle, and a small plastic bag that was ripped open.[3] In the top drawer, below the counter, police identified remnants of a white powdery substance, as well as a portable mirror with its base covered with the same white powder.[3]

Several prescription vials were found in Houston's hotel room, including for alprazolam, an antianxiety medication, two anti-inflammatory drugs, dexamethasone and prednisone, two antibiotic medicines, minocycline, for acne, and amoxicillin, a penicillin drug, as well as nystatin, for fungus, and rabeprazole, a drug prescribed for heartburn.[3]

Upstairs, police and medics were tending to Houston's body, but downstairs, celebrities wearing evening gowns and tuxedos were being dropped off by stretch limousines for Clive Davis's pre-Grammy party. [4] It wasn't long before word of Houston's death reached the arriving guests.

"I am absolutely heartbroken," Quincy Jones said when he heard the news.[5] Several guests wondered whether the party should be canceled, but Clive Davis assured them Houston would have wanted them to carry on as planned, especially since the performers had been booked months in advance. And so they did, with the atmosphere subdued and many of the guests unsure how to react.

The Autopsy

Houston's autopsy was performed the same day as the Grammys.[6] "The decedent is a forty-eight year old woman found submerged in a bathtub," Dr. Rogers, the chief of the forensic medicine division of the county of Los Angeles, wrote in the autopsy report.[6] He didn't mention that the woman was a Grammy Award–winning singer and actor.

Ten years earlier, Houston looked emaciated, but since then, she must have heeded advice to eat a healthier diet because her body was well built, muscular, and fairly well nourished.[6] A scald burn from extremely hot water was on her back, as well as small scars and several superficial abrasions all over her body, including a scar associated with breast implants.[6]

Houston's body had no tattoos. Also, no food or other foreign material was found in the mouth, upper airways, or trachea.[6] Interestingly, the upper teeth had all been replaced with a dental prosthesis that was supported by eleven dental implants.[6]

Unlike River Phoenix and John Belushi, who also abused illegal drugs and had an intact nasal septum, Houston's septum had a posterior perforation that was accompanied by a bloody purge coming from the nose. This was consistent with reports that she had been abusing cocaine and other illicit drugs over many years, most likely by nasal insuflation.[7]

Uterine leiomyoma, also known as uterine fibroids, were also identified at the autopsy.[8] These benign tumors affect women of reproductive age and can cause prolonged menstrual bleeding and severe menstrual cramps. It explained why so many packs of Midol, an over-the-counter medication to relieve symptoms of menstrual cramps, were found in Houston's hotel room.

The moderate amount of froth and fluid in Houston's lungs was a classic sign that she died by drowning.[8] The excess fluid increased the weight of her lungs, with each lung weighing twice its normal weight.[8] Also, there was evidence of mild emphysema.[8]

Of the remaining organs, the stomach was free of tablets or capsules and wasn't distended, the liver had the expected red-brown color, and its surface was smooth and soft, the kidneys were of normal weight and appearance, the bladder was unremarkable, and the thyroid and pituitary were of normal size.[8]

Cause and Manner of Death

Several drugs were found at low, therapeutic levels in Houston's blood, none of which were implicated in her death.[8] These included cyclobenzaprine, a muscle relaxant, diphenhydramine, an antihistamine, alprazolam, an antianxiety medication, ibuprofen, an over-the-counter pain killer, and marijuana.[8] Free, unmetabolized cocaine was also detected.[8] In all likelihood, Houston had consumed cocaine not long before she died because an insufficient amount of time had elapsed for the drug to be completely metabolized.[8]

Some people have speculated that alcohol must have contributed to Houston's death by making her so sedated that she slid under the water and drowned.[8] However, toxicology tests failed to find any alcohol in Houston's blood. Nevertheless, cocaethylene, a substance the liver makes by combining cocaine and alcohol, was identified.[9] This indicated that Houston drank an alcoholic beverage sometime before she died, but any alcohol that did not combine with cocaine was eliminated from her blood.[10]

The most likely explanation for why Houston died, and one with which Rogers and Sathyavagiswaran, the chief medical examiner-coroner, both agreed, is that it was an accidental drowning. Atherosclerotic heart disease due to chronic cocaine use was a contributing factor in her death. However, when I reviewed the autopsy findings related to the cardiovascular system, I noticed that although Houston's heart weight was in the normal range and free of abnormalities, there was 60 percent narrowing of the right coronary artery.[10] With that much occlusion, I wondered whether Houston had a heart attack before she drowned.

Unlike in a living person where elevated blood levels of cardiac troponin, myoglobin, cardiac enzymes, and others proteins are diagnostic indicators of a heart attack, there are no such markers in a person who has already died. Also, there was no evidence of cardiac muscle damage due to a shortage of oxygenated blood in Houston's heart.

After a thorough examination of the autopsy findings related to the cardiovascular system, I concluded there was insufficient evidence to indicate that Houston suffered a heart attack before she drowned.

Life and Career

Houston was raised in Newark, New Jersey, one of the oldest cities in the United States. The city is the largest and second-most racially diverse city in New Jersey, a state from which many famous people had originated, including Frank Sinatra, Ice-T, Meryl Streep, Jerry Lewis of Dean Martin and Jerry Lewis comedy team fame, and Norman Schwarzkopf, the United States Army general who led the coalition forces in the Gulf War.[11]

There was never any doubt Houston was destined to become a singer. Her mother, Cissy Houston, was a famous gospel singer, and her cousin, Dion Warwick, was a legendary singer who teamed up with Burt Bacharach to sing "Walk on By" and "I Say a Little Prayer."[11]

When she was eleven years old, Houston began to sing as a soloist in the junior gospel choir at the New Hope Baptist Church. "I think I knew then that [my ability to sing] was an infectious thing that God had given me," Houston told Diane Sawyer in a 2002 interview.[12] By the time she was fifteen, Houston toured nightclubs with her mother and sang backup vocals on Chaka Khan's 1978 hit "I'm Every Woman," as well as for Lou Rawls and Jermaine Jackson.[13]

When Clive Davis offered to sign Houston to a recording contract, she immediately accepted.[13] She was just nineteen at the time, but their collaboration continued until her death.

At twenty-one, Houston's debut album, *Whitney Houston*, became the biggest-selling album by a debut artist. One of the album's songs, "Saving All My Love for You," won a Grammy Award for Best Pop Female Vocal Performance.[13] *Rolling Stone* magazine labeled

Houston "one of the most exciting new voices in years" and concluded "Whitney Houston is obviously headed for stardom."[14] Under Clive Davis's guidance, Houston's singing career began to soar.

Super Bowl XXV was on Sunday, January 21, 1991, just ten days after the first Persian Gulf War began. One hundred and fifteen million people nationwide waited to view the televised game. Everybody was excited to see the New York Giants play the Buffalo Bills at Tampa Stadium in Tampa, Florida. Although neither team had come out of their locker room yet, the color guards were already on the field.

Frank Gifford, the former New York Giants halfback and an inductee into the Pro Football Hall of Fame, made the announcement. "And now, to honor America, especially the brave men and women serving our nation in the Persian Gulf and throughout the world, please join in the singing of our national anthem ... sung by Grammy Award–winner Whitney Houston."[15]

A deafening cheer rose from the stands as the twenty-seven-year-old Houston stepped up to the platform, wearing a white tracksuit with red and blue accents, white Nike shoes, and with her hair held back with a bandanna.[16] Backed by the Florida Orchestra, a huge smile across her face, Houston was ready to sing the national anthem in front of over seventy-three thousand fans and a worldwide audience of 750 million people.[17]

"The Star-Spangled Banner" was not an easy song to sing. From the moment Houston opened her mouth, however, the audience knew she had put her personal mark on the music. And when she finished singing, Houston raised her arms in a wide arc and pumped her fists in the air, surrounded by a thunderous noise as the public expressed an overwhelming feeling of patriotism and pride in the United States and all that it represented.

"If you were there, you could feel the intensity," Houston later said.[18] "The love coming out of the stands was incredible."[18] It wasn't only magical, it was inspiring.

Inundated by phone calls about Houston's interpretation of the national anthem, and the song being aired by hundreds of radio stations, Arista Records released a record of the performance on February 12, 1991.[19] The video followed five days later. "The Star-Spangled Banner" sung by Houston quickly became one of her top-selling hits.[20]

Houston would soon attain even greater acclaim with her acting debut in *The Bodyguard* and the release of the movie's soundtrack.[21] "I wanted to do some acting, but I never thought I'd be costarring with Kevin Costner," she told *Rolling Stone* magazine about her involvement in *The Bodyguard*.[22] "It took me two years to decide to do it."[22] The film became the second-highest grossing film worldwide, making more than $400 million, and the soundtrack won a Grammy Award for Album of the Year and was the best-selling soundtrack, with more than forty-two million copies sold worldwide.[23]

Within ten years, Houston's career, which until then was in a steep, upward trajectory, declined to unprecedented lows as her life unraveled and spiraled out of control.

After her second album was released, Houston won her second Grammy for Best Female Pop Vocal Performance, as well as two American Music Awards and a Soul Train Music Award. In 1991, she married R&B singer Bobby Brown. The marriage, which lasted fourteen years, was dubbed "the most tumultuous relationship in music history."[24]

By 1997, Houston had won numerous other awards and appeared in two more films, *Waiting to Exhale* and *The Preacher's Wife*, as well as in a made-for-television remake of *Cinderella*. She released five more albums and starred in a remake of the film *Sparkle*, but unfortunately, she would never get to see the film released.

Sometime toward the end of the twentieth century, Houston's behavior dramatically changed.[25] She would often forget the lyrics to some of her most famous songs, would be late for interviews and photo shoots, and would cancel concerts and appearances on talk shows, even missing performing for her mentor, Clive Davis, when he was inducted into the Rock and Roll Hall of Fame.[26] Rumors of drug use were widespread. In 2000, marijuana was discovered in Houston's luggage at an airport in Hawaii.[27] "It wasn't Bobby Brown who introduced her to drugs," Houston's former sister-in-law told *Newsweek* magazine.[28] "Drugs were around her for years before she met Bobby and continued after he left."[28]

At the Michael Jackson: 30th Anniversary Special at Madison Square Garden in 2001, Houston was shockingly thin, which only further flamed speculation that she was abusing drugs.[29] When Diane Sawyer confronted her about allegations of drug use, Houston replied, "Crack is cheap. I make too much money to ever smoke crack." However, she acknowledged she drank alcohol to excess, smoked marijuana, and abused cocaine and drugs.[30] In 2009, Houston told Oprah Winfrey that she and Brown would "lace marijuana with rock cocaine" and admitted that while she abused drugs before making *The Bodyguard*, her drug use became much heavier after the film was released.[31]

Houston attended a drug rehabilitation program on multiple occasions but would always return to drugs after she was released.[32] While she tried to reinvigorate her career in the late 2000s, reviews of her Nothing

But Love World Tour were mediocre, and her tribute performance to Dionne Warwick at a pre-Grammy gala in 2011 was poorly received.[33]

Conclusion

The *Guinness Book of World Records* lists Houston as music's "most awarded female artist of all time" with at least 411 awards.[34] "Her life was full of betrayal and disappointment," Kevin Macdonald, director of the Houston family-sanctioned documentary, *Whitney*, said after Houston's death.[35] She "was hopeless giving interviews, always surface-level, and she never wrote her own songs. So it's really about the nonverbal message she's imparting."[36]

Pat Houston, executor of the Houston estate, told a reporter, "Everybody loved her, but no one would step up and help her," referring to Houston's drug addiction.[37]

Before Houston's body was laid to rest, it was returned one last time to the New Hope Baptist Church, the place from which Houston rose to fame.[38] Her family and friends mourned Houston in a four-hour televised celebration of her life and career.[39] Later, on the way to the cemetery, a crowd of about one hundred fans lined the street as the procession, with the driver of the gold hearse crying behind the wheel and a photo of Houston posted on the window, carried Houston's body and brought it to Westfield, New Jersey, for burial.[40]

Houston's legacy was marred by drug use, a decline in the quality of her musical performances, and a tragic end to an otherwise magical life. But her career spanned nearly thirty years, most of which were remarkable and hugely entertaining.

"The Whitney Houston I knew was still wondering if I'm good enough," Kevin Costner, Houston's co-star in *The Bodyguard*, said at her funeral. "It was what made her great, and what caused her to stumble at the end."[40]

Houston's music will live long after her death, almost exactly fifty three years after "the day the music died" when Buddy Holly, the Big Bopper, and Ritchie Valens died in a plane crash.[41] Sales of Houston's songs and albums neared one million copies just one day after fans learned of her death. Her biggest hit, "I Will Always Love You," was downloaded 195,000 times in one week, up from three thousand the previous week.[42] Five years after Houston's death, total sales of her albums continued to climb, reaching more than 3,700,000.[43]

"You wait for a voice like that for a lifetime," Clive Davis said at Houston's funeral.[44] "You wait for a face like that, a smile like that, a presence like that for a lifetime. When one person embodies it all, it takes your breath away."[45]

Recalling Houston, Neil Portnow, president of the National Academy of Recording Arts and Sciences, said she was "one of the greatest pop singers of all time who leaves behind a robust musical soundtrack."[46]

CHAPTER 19

Philip Seymour Hoffman

Died February 2, 2014

On Sunday, February 2, 2014, Philip Seymour Hoffman, an Oscar-winning character actor, was supposed to pick up his kids at Mimi O'Donnell's apartment, but he didn't show up.[1] David Bar Katz, one of Hoffman's friends, and Isabella Wing-Davey, Hoffman's assistant, went to Hoffman's apartment to check on him. But when they opened the door, they found Hoffman lying dead on the bathroom floor, clad in shorts and a T-shirt with his glasses still on his head and a syringe stuck in his left arm.[2] He was forty-six years old. When police arrived to investigate, they found fifty small bags labeled "Ace of Spades," which they believed contained heroin.[2]

The Autopsy

The autopsy and toxicology reports were unavailable for review. However, the New York Medical Examiner's Office announced that Hoffman had heroin, cocaine, benzodiazepine tranquilizers, and amphetamine in his blood.[3]

Cause and Manner of Death

In college, Hoffman had engaged in "advanced drinking and drugging," as he later recalled.[4] He had used "anything I could get my hands on … I liked it all," he said.[5] When he was twenty-two years old, he checked himself into a rehab facility.[6] "It made me worried if I was going to get to do the kind of things I wanted to do in my life," Hoffman declared in a 2006 interview.[7]

For twenty-three years, Hoffman abstained from drugs and alcohol, but in May 2013, he relapsed into snorting heroin.[8] "He started having a drink or two without it seeming a big deal," O'Donnell, Hoffman's longtime partner and mother of his three children, said, "but the moment drugs came into play … he told me that it was just this one time, and that it wouldn't happen again."[9]

Hoffman checked himself into rehab for a second time, but this time, "Within a day or two of returning, he started using [heroin] again," said O'Donnell.[9] "You're going to die. That's what happens with heroin," she told him.[9] Hoffman's addiction was too much for O'Donnell to deal with, and soon, Hoffman moved out of their Greenwich Village home and into an apartment, only two blocks away.[10] Sometimes he would be seen disheveled and drinking alone in bars.[10]

A week before he died, Hoffman called a reporter, sounding barely awake and incoherent, forgetful, and slurring his words.[11] "The addiction was bigger than either of us," O'Donnell told *Vogue* magazine.[12] *I can't fix this*, she thought. "It was the moment that I let go."[12]

A spokesperson from the New York Medical Examiner's Office announced that Hoffman died of acute mixed drug intoxication caused by heroin, cocaine, benzodiazepine tranquilizers, and amphetamine and that the manner of death was an accident.[13]

Like many addicts, Hoffman may have been under the false impression that when stimulants were taken together with depressants, the toxic effects of the drugs would cancel each other out. However, in fact, the stimulant effects had undoubtedly dissipated much sooner than the depressant effects, and as a result, Hoffman died from respiratory depression and cardiotoxicity caused by the delayed heroin overdose in combination with benzodiazepine sedative drugs.

Life and Career

Born in Fairport, a suburb of Rochester, New York, Hoffman saw the play *All My Sons* when he was twelve years old and was completely transformed by the experience.[14] "I was changed, permanently changed," he told the *New York Times*.[15] "It was like a miracle to me."

In his midteens, instead of trying out for the school baseball team, Hoffman got involved in acting because he was attracted to a girl. "I perceived myself as not attractive," he recalled, but "there was this beautiful girl. I had a huge crush on her, and she acted. It seemed like something worth giving up baseball for."[15] He played the part of Radar in the school production of *MASH*. By his senior year, he was given the role of Willy Loman in *Death of a Salesman*.[16]

When he was seventeen, Hoffman attended the New York State Summer School of the Arts in Saratoga Springs.[17] Before enrolling at New York University's Tisch School of the Arts, where he received a degree in drama, Hoffman spent a summer at the Circle in the

Square Theater School in Manhattan.[18] After graduating from New York University, Hoffman appeared in off Broadway theater productions.

In 1991, Hoffman made his on-screen debut in a segment of the television program *Law & Order*. Bit parts in independent films soon followed.[19] After auditioning five times, Hoffman succeeded in getting the part of a prep school student in *Scent of a Woman*.[20] His performance won him the attention of film critics. [20] "It was pure joy to get to do the work," Hoffman said, referring to his villainous character in the film.[20] "If I hadn't gotten into that film, I wouldn't be where I am today."[21]

By the time he was awarded the 2005 Oscar for Best Actor for his role in *Capote*, Hoffman had appeared in many other memorable roles: as a storm chaser in *Twister*, a mobster in *The Getaway*, a policeman in *Nobody's Fool*, as well as in *Boogie Nights*, *The Big Lebowski*, *Magnolia*, and *The Talented Mr. Ripley*.[22] Between 2007 and 2012, he received three more Oscar nominations for his performances as a CIA agent in *Charlie Wilson's War* (2007), a priest under suspicion in *Doubt* (2008), and a cult leader in *The Master* (2012).[22]

Hoffman was also very active in the theatre, appearing in three Broadway shows, all of which earned him Tony Award nominations—*True West* (2000), *Long Day's*

Journey into Night (2003), and *Death of a Salesman* (2012).[23] His most challenging role was in *Long Day's Journey into Night*.[24] "That nearly killed me," Hoffman told the *New York Times*.[25] Robert Falls, director of the play, agreed. "He just brought every fiber of his being to the stage."[25]

Before he died, Hoffman had completed filming nearly all his scenes in *The Hunger Games: Mockingjay—Part 2*. His two remaining scenes were rewritten after his death, and the film was released in November 2015.

Hoffman was an actor who was admired by his peers for his talent, intensity, and commitment to his craft. When he heard that Hoffman died, Matt Singer, editor of *The Dissolve,* said, "He was great in great movies like *The Master* and he was great in bad movies like *Along Came Polly*."[26] Scott Tobias of *The Dissolve* agreed. "He was the most electric actor of his generation."[26] O'Donnell reflected on her and Hoffman's time together, saying Hoffman was "a sweet and gentle and loving man ... a sensitive person."[27]

Despite all the accolades, Hoffman remained insecure, both about himself and his performances. "A lot of people describe me as chubby ... or stocky ... I'm waiting for somebody to say I'm at least cute," he said. "But nobody has."[28] In a 2005 *Rolling Stone* magazine interview, he claimed, "No one knows me. No one understands me."[28]

Conclusion

Like many entertainers, Hoffman was addicted to drugs. "From the beginning, [he] was very frank about his addictions," said O'Donnell.[29] When we first started dating, "he told me that, as much as he loved me, if I used drugs, it would be a deal breaker."[29] Ironically, for some unexplained reason, and after twenty-three years of being drug-free, Hoffman again began to abuse illicit drugs. "I hate to ascribe [his] relapse after two decades to any one thing, or even to a series of things," O'Donnell said.[29] "Lots of people go through difficult life events. Only addicts start taking drugs to blunt the pain of them."[29]

Hoffman left behind a career of fifty-five theater, television, and film performances. And yet he was the toughest on himself. "Acting is so difficult for me that … unless I reach the expectations I have of myself, I'm unhappy," Hoffman said.[30] Todd Louiso, a friend of Hoffman and a writer-director, told *Rolling Stone* magazine, "He channeled that addictive personality into his work."[30] But as Hoffman became more successful and his stature as an actor grew, "The thing he hated most was the loss of anonymity," said O'Donnell.[31] Hoffman "was never comfortable with celebrity … [but he] was endlessly generous with his time and energy and money." [32] Nevertheless, as good and as generous as Hoffman was, it was impossible for O'Donnell to stay in a relationship with an active addict. "It feels like being boiled in oil," she said.[32] When Hoffman died, as O'Donnell had rightly predicted would happen, "There was no sense of peace or relief, just ferocious pain and overwhelming loss."[32]

CHAPTER 20
Robin Williams
Died August 11, 2014

ON THE EVENING of August 10, 2014, Robin Williams, an extremely funny comedian and actor, placed several of his designer wrist watches in a sock and drove them to a friend's house, approximately two miles away. Afraid they would be stolen, he gave the watches to his friend for safekeeping, a behavior that was consistent with Williams's symptoms of paranoia. [1] After he returned home at about 10:30 p.m., Williams and his wife, who slept in separate bedrooms, retired for the night. [2]

Williams went into his wife's bedroom several times during the night, at one time taking his iPad out of the room. [3] The next morning, his wife awoke and, seeing Williams's bedroom door locked, assumed he was still asleep, so she went to run some errands. When she returned, she became concerned because Williams's door was still closed.[4] She slipped a note under the door and asked if Williams was all right, but she received no reply.[4] Eventually, Williams's assistant gained access to the room and found Williams lying unresponsive on the floor.[5]

When paramedics arrived, they found Williams in a sitting position next to the closet door with a black nylon belt tied around his neck.[6] Near the bed was a chair, and on the chair were two prescription vials containing quetiapine and mirtazapine, two antipsychotic drugs Williams had been taking to combat his depression.[6] A pocketknife, which Williams's wife confirmed was her husband's, was also found on the chair. It had dried blood on both sides of the blade.[6] Other items identified in Williams's room included an iPad and a cell phone, neither of which provided any evidence that Williams had phone conversations about suicide.[6] And in the bathroom, paramedics found a damp white washcloth with reddish stains, later identified as blood.[6]

Williams was pronounced dead at noon, but he probably died sometime around midnight the previous night because partially digested food was found in his stomach, consistent with remnants of his last meal.[6]

The Autopsy

Williams's autopsy was performed by Dr. Joseph I. Cohen, a graduate of the Medical College of Wisconsin and the chief forensic pathologist of Marin County in Northern California.[7] Cohen identified a nine-inch vertical scar on Williams's upper chest, undoubtedly from his recent heart surgery, as well as a three-and-a-half-inch scar on the lower right quadrant of Williams's abdomen from a previous surgery to remove his appendix, which was absent.[8] A tattoo was present on Williams's left hip.[8]

It was immediately obvious that Williams had committed suicide and that his death was a result of asphyxiation. He was found in his bedroom with a belt tied around his neck, and the bruising and ligature marks on his neck were consistent with hanging.[8] Alcohol was not implicated in Williams's death, as none was detected in his blood. Nor was foul play suspected, as there were no skull fractures or hemorrhages under Williams's scalp or in his brain.[9]

I was very distressed, however, by how determined Williams was to end his life. Besides the evidence he hanged himself, there were approximately ten fresh, superficial, and slightly oozing wounds on his left wrist. [10] The cuts were self-inflicted, which was confirmed by DNA analysis establishing blood on Williams's pocketknife as his own.[10] I was convinced Williams had tried to cut his wrists before he hanged himself, and the only reason he didn't bleed to death was because he had failed to cut any of the major vessels.

Williams's cardiovascular system appeared to have been functioning well. While his heart was markedly enlarged and a risk factor for sudden death, it's unlikely Williams had suffered an arrhythmia before he died.[10] Also, his new aortic valve and his repaired mitral valve were both free of clots, and the major vessels of his heart were only minimally narrowed by plaque, so that his risk for a heart attack was low.[10]

Like Michael Jackson who died before him, Williams also had a prostate that was slightly enlarged and nodular, with no evidence of cancer.[10] It explained why a bottle of finasteride, a drug that shrinks the size of the prostate and reduces symptoms associated with an enlarged prostate, was discovered in his home.[10]

Dense tau protein positive neurofibrillary tangles were identified in the anterior hippocampus and temporal cortex, areas of the brain responsible for cognitive function, mood control, and emotion.[11] These abnormalities, often seen in patients suffering from

Parkinson-like tremors, were a clear indication of the cause of Williams's cognitive decline.[11] Also, the right substantia nigra of the brain, an area that plays a critical role in modulating motor movement, appeared pale in comparison to the left.[12] However, the most prominent features in Williams's brain were the presence of Lewy bodies, abnormal protein deposits that disrupt the brain's normal function, and a 30 to 40 percent degeneration of neurons, the highway in the central nervous system that carries electrical impulses from the brain to the rest of the body.[13] Together, these findings supported a diagnosis of diffuse Lewy body dementia, a progressive form of dementia that frequently presents with Parkinson's-like motor symptoms, depression, and hallucinations.[14]

Of Williams's remaining organs, the lungs were well inflated, smooth, and glistening, the liver was smooth with a normal red-brown color, the kidneys had slight congestion but were otherwise unremarkable, the adrenals had some congestion, and the pituitary, pancreas, and thyroid were all normal.[15]

Cause and Manner of Death

Toxicology analysis failed to detect any drugs of abuse in Williams's blood. However, low, therapeutic amounts of two antipsychotic drugs, mirtazapine and levodopa, both of which had been prescribed for Williams's depression, were identified.[15] Also detected were caffeine and theobromine, a metabolite of caffeine.[15] This, along with the absence of needle tracks on Williams's arms, supported the claim that Williams had been drug-free for many years.[16]

After I reviewed all the relevant records, I agreed with the coroner's conclusion that the cause of Williams's death was asphyxiation and that the manner of death was a suicide.

Life and Career

Early research has shown that approximately 85 percent of comedians come from low socioeconomic backgrounds.[17] However, that wasn't the case with Williams. An only child, Williams grew up in an affluent neighborhood in Illinois.[18] His mother was a former model, and his father, a Ford Motor Company senior executive.[18] Shy, overweight, and bullied in school, Williams often played by himself with toy soldiers, taking on different voices for each one.[19] He credited his early interest in comedy to his mother, who, unlike his very intense father, had a sense of humor.[20]

Williams briefly studied political science at Claremont Men's College, but after taking a course in theatre at College of Marin, he accepted a three-year scholarship to study theatre at the Julliard School of Performing Arts in New York City under the famous actor and producer John Houseman.[21] However, after only two years, Williams left Julliard because, as one of his teachers told him, there was nothing more Julliard could teach him.[21] Instead of acting in Shakespearean plays, Williams decided to try his luck as a stand-up comedian in California.[21]

It was while performing at the Comedy Club in Los Angeles that Williams was discovered by George Schlatter, a television producer, to appear in a revival of the 1960s show *Laugh In*.[21] The show didn't run long, but Williams's performance was noticed by entertainment agents, and he was asked to appear on *The Richard Pryor Show*.[21] By coincidence, Gary Marshall was looking for an actor to play Mork, an alien from Ork, who was sent to investigate the culture on Earth for a dream segment on *Happy Days*.[21] When Marshall saw Williams on *The Richard Prior Show*, he asked him to audition for the part. Williams was selected when he sat on his head at the audition with his rear facing up in the air.[21] Marshall said Williams was the only alien who auditioned.[21]

Viewers were so taken with Williams's performance on *Happy Days* that *Mork & Mindy* was created in 1970 as a spin-off to give Williams a vehicle to display his uniquely zany brand of comedy.[21] Seeing Williams wearing a T-shirt and multicolored suspenders was mind-boggling.[21] How can anyone ever forget "Na-nu, Na-nu!"—the famous words uttered by Mork?[22]

Williams' improvisational style and ad-libbing were fresh and turned situational comedy completely on its head. He made talking gibberish normal, and the audience loved it. "I'm a test tube baby," Mork said in the first episode.[23] "My father was an eye dropper, the scum. He ran away and left my mom. Ran away with a bottle of nose drops."[24] A new star was born!

It is said that Williams ad-libbed so much on the show that the producers left gaps in the scripts and simply noted "Mork can go off here."[24] *Mork & Mindy* became a huge hit in part because Williams wasn't only exceptionally funny, he was also unpredictable.[24]

In 1980, Williams made his feature film debut in *Popeye*, playing the spinach-loving sailor whose love interest, Olive Oyl, was played by Shelley Duvall.[24] His performance in *Popeye* was followed by comedic roles in *The World According to Garp* and *The Survivors*.[24] However, it was his 1994 dramatic role as a Russian saxophone player who defects to America to work at Bloomingdale's, a New York department store, in the film *Moscow on the Hudson* that brought Williams recognition for his acting talent.[25] Success in *Moscow on the Hudson* led to other dramatic roles, including in *Good Morning Vietnam*, *Dead Poets Society*, and *The Fisher King*.[26] Williams received Academy Award nominations for Best Actor in a Leading Role in all three of the films before winning an Oscar for Best Actor in a Supporting Role in *Good Will Hunting*.[26] Other memorable films included *Hook, Aladdin, Mrs. Doubtfire,* and *Night at the Museum*.[26]

Throughout his career, Williams won many awards and accolades, but his success came at a heavy price. His indulgence in alcohol and drugs, which began while performing in *Mork & Mindy*, continued to escalate with his increasing fame.[27] While he quit drinking alcohol in the 1980s, when his first wife became pregnant, "cocaine was a place to hide," Williams told *People* magazine.[28] Unlike in other people, "cocaine slowed me down."[28] However, when his good friend John Belushi died from a cocaine overdose, Williams abruptly quit abusing cocaine.[29]

In March 2009, Williams began to experience shortness of breath for which he underwent heart surgery at the Cleveland Clinic.[30] During the three and a half hours of his surgery, Williams's aortic valve was replaced, his mitral valve was repaired, and his irregular heartbeat was corrected.[30] Then, in 2011, Williams exhibited neuromuscular symptoms and tremors for which he ultimately was diagnosed with Parkinson's disease.[31] There were also periods when he couldn't remember his lines, as well as moments of confusion, visual disturbances, and symptoms of depression that included paranoia, delusions, compulsiveness, and anxiety.[32] Williams's doctors assured him that drugs were available to control his tremors, but they couldn't offer him anything to slow down the loss of his cognitive abilities.[33] As if these health problems weren't enough, Williams's new TV show, *The Crazy Ones*, was cancelled in 2014 after only one season.[34] According to his wife, the depression and slow, progressive decline of Williams's mental abilities affected him immensely.[35] He "was losing his mind and he was aware of it," she said.[35]

I have no doubt Williams was despondent in the days leading up to his death. An examination of the browsing history on his iPad revealed he had researched his medications, so he must have been aware of his rapidly deteriorating cognitive and physical abilities.[36] It isn't unreasonable to conclude, therefore, that Williams learned that with time, his condition would only deteriorate further.

Williams relied on his wit, intellect, and physicality to deliver some of his funniest moments on stage and on television. He may have felt lost without the ability to continue to do so. "I don't know how to be funny [anymore]," he told Cheri Minns, a member of the makeup crew during the filming of *Night at the Museum: Secret of the Tomb*.[37]

"I never heard him afraid like that before," Billy Crystal, Williams's close friend, said when he heard that Williams was diagnosed with Parkinson's.[38] "Think of it this way," Crystal said when the autopsy report was released, "the speed at which the comedy came is the speed at which the terror came … I can't imagine living like that."[38] Williams's wife agreed. "He hated that he could not find the words he wanted in conversations." [39] In a 2016 editorial in the scientific journal *Neurology*, she wrote, "His loss of basic reasoning just added to his growing confusion … Can you imagine the pain he felt as he experienced himself disintegrating?"[39]

Conclusion

It's important to distinguish between what led Williams to commit suicide and the cause of his cognitive and physical symptoms. While a medical explanation was provided for Williams's mental and physical deterioration when a diagnosis of diffuse Lewy body dementia was finally made, it would be mere speculation to conclude that it would have made a difference had Williams learned of his diagnosis while he was still alive.[39] "He would surely [have] become one of the most famous test subjects of new medicines and ongoing medical trials," his wife wrote in *Neurology*.[39]

In a case study published in the scientific journal *Trends in Psychiatry and Psychotherapy*, Hassaan Tohid of the Center for Mind & Brain at the University of California at Davis noted Williams had suffered from major depression, alcoholism, drug abuse, and Lewy body dementia, and had financial problems and serious relationship issues, leading to multiple divorces.[40] With the exception of Lewy body dementia, Tohid concluded, "a combination of all these factors, or the comorbid condition of such severity, even though not apparent to the world, ultimately led to [Williams's] suicide."[40] But "whether Lewy body dementia can trigger suicide, and whether it contributed to his suicide, is still a matter of debate."[40]

Williams was not only a comedian with many unique talents who broke barriers, he was an award-winning and accomplished actor. Slowly losing his mental capacity and his gift for comedy, he knew that without his mental faculties, there was only despair to look forward to. "You're only given a little spark of madness," he once said.[41] "If you lose that, you're nothing."

CHAPTER 21

Joan Rivers

Died September 4, 2014

JOAN RIVERS, THE octogenarian, highly successful comedian, had a history of acid reflux disease and had been complaining for some time of being hoarse.[1] She had finally scheduled an esophagogastroduodenoscopy (EGD), a minor elective medical procedure in which a thin scope with a light and a camera at its tip is used to look inside the area between the throat and small bowel. [2] It was to be performed by Dr. Lawrence B. Cohen, the director of Yorkville Endoscopy in New York.[2] The clinic, a licensed outpatient surgery center on Manhattan's East Side, was one of a growing number of medical centers that had replaced hospital operating rooms for minor surgeries.[3]

The evening before her EGD, Rivers was at the Laurie Beechman Theatre, trying out some of her new material. [4] Reading off cue cards, she joked about her mortality. Her words turned out to be prophetic. "I could go at any moment," she told the approximately one hundred fans who had gathered to see her hour-long show.[4] "I could lay here and go over ... and it would be in the papers and you all could look at each other and say I was there the night Joan Rivers passed," she said.[4]

When Rivers arrived at the clinic on the morning of August 28, 2014, she was accompanied by Dr. Gwen Korovin, a prominent ear, nose, and throat specialist whose celebrity patients included Ariana Grande, Celine Dion, and Joel Gray, among others.[5] Korovin planned to perform a nasolaryngoscopy, a diagnostic examination of the voice box and vocal cords that was done by passing a thin scope through Rivers's nose.[5]

The medical procedures were to begin at about nine o'clock in the morning. Rivers's vital signs at the time were within normal limits. Prior to conducting the procedures, Rivers was sedated with propofol, the same general anesthetic that had been administered to Michael Jackson the day he died.

After Rivers was anesthetized, Korovin attempted to perform the nasolaryngoscopy; however, she had difficulty and aborted the procedure.[6] About seven minutes later, Rivers's blood pressure began to significantly drop, and it continued to do so over the next seventeen minutes.[6] Nevertheless, Cohen went ahead with the EGD. When he was finished, Korovin again tried to perform the nasolaryngoscopy, and this time, she was successful.[6] It was then that Rivers experienced laryngospasm, a problematic reflex that often occurs under general anesthesia.[7] Her breathing soon stopped, and she went into cardiac arrest.[7] Attempts were immediately made to resuscitate her with epinephrine and atropine, two drugs that stimulate the heart, but although successful, it took much too long.[8]

Rivers was transferred to Mount Sinai Hospital where she was put in intensive care. A week later, after having suffered significant brain damage from a lack of oxygen, she was taken off life support and died.[8]

The Autopsy

Since Rivers died in a hospital following therapeutic complications from a routine medical procedure, an autopsy and toxicology tests were not conducted.

Cause and Manner of Death

New York City's medical examiner concluded that Rivers died after suffering a "predictable complication of medical therapy."[9] The cause of death was "anoxic encephalopathy due to hypoxic arrest during laryngoscopy and upper gastrointestinal endoscopy with propofol sedation for evaluation of voice changes and gastroesophageal reflux disease."[9] In other words, Rivers died from a lack of oxygen to the brain during performance of a routine, minor outpatient medical procedure.

A month after Rivers's medical emergency at the Yorkville Endoscopy, the clinic was reviewed by New York's Centers for Medicare & Medicaid Services, Department of Health and Human Services.[10] In November 2014, the New York Centers' report was finally released. It found the clinic had failed to ensure that services were provided in a manner that protected the health and safety of all patients."[10] The report further concluded Cohen had failed to identify Rivers's deteriorating vital signs and to provide timely intervention during the EGD procedure. Shockingly, the report noted Cohen had taken cell phone photos of Rivers while she was sedated.[10] As for Korovin, the other doctor who was involved in Rivers's care, the report concluded she was not a member of the clinic's medical staff, did not have privileges at the clinic, and didn't have an informed consent to conduct the nasolaryngoscopy. Surprisingly, Rivers's body weight wasn't recorded, so it may not have been used to determine the dose of propofol. Also, the amount of the administered anesthetic was inconsistently reported in the medical records.

Propofol anesthesia is known to be associated with hypotension, so it undoubtedly was responsible for the drop in Rivers's blood pressure.[11] That may explain why Cohen didn't seem concerned when he went ahead with the EGD anyway. Ironically, propofol has also been reported to relieve laryngospasm.[12] Most likely, Rivers's laryngospasm was a normal response to the procedures that occurs in some patients. However, death under such minor, elective procedures is very rare.

The risk of laryngospasm during anesthesia is increased by a combination of anesthetic and surgery-related factors such as a patient's age, intensity of the anesthesia—light anesthesia may lead to a predisposition to trigger laryngospasm—and treatment of the airways, such as the placement of a nasogastric tube.[13] Rivers was eighty-one years old, so she was at a greater risk of laryngospasm. Also, since her weight was not recorded, it's possible she wasn't administered sufficient anesthetic to cause deep sedation.[14]

In her article in *Modern Health Care* magazine, Sabriya Rice noted older adults are at a greater risk of surgical complications.[15] "Not all ambulatory surgical centers are staffed to handle a crisis ... [whereas] ... in a hospital, emergency teams are able to respond rapidly," said Rice.[15] It was certainly true with Rivers who had to be transported to Mount Sinai Hospital to receive the medical attention she needed after she stopped breathing and had gone into cardiac arrest.

It's possible Rivers's medical emergency at Yorkville Endoscopy could have been prevented. "[Anytime] you operate [on] a person's vocal cords, you run the risk of [inducing] laryngospasm paralysis ..., which will lead to respiratory failure if not corrected immediately," internist Dr. Simon Murray said.[16] Dr. Renuka Bankulla, the anesthesiologist at Yorkville Endoscopy, had cautioned Cohen against proceeding with the EGD after she noticed Rivers's vocal cords were extremely swollen, but he ignored her pleadings.[17] "You're being paranoid," he was reported to have told her and then proceeded with the EGD anyway. Soon thereafter, Korovin performed the nasolaryngoscopy.[17] Chaos then ensued when Rivers suffered laryngospasm and went into cardiac arrest.[18]

It has been reported that 61 percent of people who suffer laryngospasm experience hypoxia, a lack of oxygen to the brain.[19] Rivers was one of those people.

It didn't take long after the report of the New York's Centers for Medicare & Medicaid Services was released for Melissa, Rivers's daughter, to file a multimillion-dollar lawsuit against Yorkville Endoscopy and all the physicians and anesthesiologists who were responsible for her mother's care.[20] By the time the case settled, Cohen had already resigned as clinic director. Nevertheless, the doctors accepted responsibility for their actions, and a substantial financial settlement was paid.[21]

Life and Career

The daughter of Russian Jewish immigrants, Rivers was raised in Larchmont, a suburb of New York City. [22] After attending Barnard College, where she acted in several productions, Rivers worked in the publicity department of Lord & Taylor department store and then as a fashion coordinator for Bond men's clothing stores. [23] She married the son of the Bond stores' merchandiser, but the marriage was annulled after six months.[23]

Rivers returned to her true passion, performing in front of a live audience.[24] She acted in several small plays but quickly realized that her talent was more suited to comedy.[24] Over the next seven years, she did stand-up comedy at various New York City comedy clubs and coffeehouses.[24]

"I was brought up seven times to the *Carson* show, and they rejected me each time," Rivers recalled of her early auditions for *The Tonight Show Starring Johnny Carson*.[25] Eventually, the producers of the show allowed her to sit on the couch next to Carson, not as a comedienne but as a "funny girl writer," before she made her official debut performance in 1965.[26] "You're going to be a star," Carson told Rivers when he couldn't help laughing at her routine.[27] An instant hit, Rivers never looked back.

Over the next eighteen years, Rivers's career continued to advance. She was a headliner in Las Vegas and on television, had a Grammy-nominated comedy album, a best-selling book, *The Life and Hard Times of Heidi Abromowitz*, and was on *The Tonight Show* more than seventy-five times, including as a permanent guest host.[28] "[Carson] handed me my career," Rivers said of her mentor.[28] "I gave him my unwavering loyalty. I never wanted to do anything to hurt that man."[28]

By the mid-1980s, after turning down multiple offers from other networks, Rivers's contract with NBC was renewed for only one year.[28] It was the first hint Rivers had that she probably wouldn't be selected to replace Carson when he retired as host of *The Tonight Show*. Her suspicion was confirmed when she saw an NBC interoffice memo that named potential successors to Carson, but her name was not included on the list.[28]

When negotiations with NBC broke down, Rivers signed with Fox to host *The Late Show Starring Joan Rivers*.[28] Carson was furious that she didn't consult with him before she made her decision. Rivers claimed she called him twice and that he hung up on her each time. Nevertheless, from that day forward, Carson never spoke to Rivers again.[29]

The Late Show Starring Joan Rivers lasted less than a year.[30] Carson let it be known that anyone who appeared on Rivers's show would be blackballed from *The Tonight Show*, which made booking celebrities on the Joan Rivers's show almost impossible.[31]

In August 1987, Rivers's second husband, who was also her manager, committed suicide by overdosing on diazepam, a sedative and hypnotic drug.[32] Rivers had hoped Carson would contact her to show his respect, but he never did. After the funeral, Rivers discovered her husband had made some bad investments and had left her $37 million in debt.[33] Moreover, no one in the entertainment world wanted to hire her.[33] A single mom, she was desperate.

Rivers's feud with Carson was not the first time a comedian had a public feud with a powerful television host. In 1964, Jackie Mason, the very funny comedian with a heavy Jewish accent, appeared on the *Ed Sullivan Show* the same night President Johnson was scheduled to speak.[34] Sullivan, standing off camera, motioned with his fingers that Mason should wrap up his monologue. [34] When Mason saw Sullivan's finger gestures, he mimicked them in his act.[34] Thinking Mason was giving him "the finger," Sullivan was incensed and immediately terminated Mason's contract.[34] Mason sued Sullivan, a suit he eventually won.[34] Sullivan apologized on the air, but the damage had already been done.[34] It took fifteen years for Mason's career to recover from the dispute.[35]

Determined to move on, Rivers designed and sold her own line of costume jewelry and other products on QVC. She launched her own syndicated daytime TV show in 1989, for which she won an Emmy Award and was honored with a star on Hollywood's Walk of Fame. She also cowrote and starred in *Sally Marr ... and Her Escorts* in 1994, for which she was nominated for a Tony Award for best actress.[36] In addition, Rivers served as host of *Live from the Red Carpet* and *Fashion Police*, had her own TV reality show *Joan & Melissa: Joan Knows Best?,* published a dozen books, including *I Hate Everyone ... Starting with Me* and *Diary of a Mad Diva*, and performed stand-up comedy routines several times a year.[36]

In 2014, forty-nine years after her first appearance on *The Tonight Show* and long after Carson died, Rivers returned to *The Tonight Show*.[37] By then, Jimmy Fallon was host.[37] "It's about time," Rivers joked. "I've been sitting in a taxi outside NBC with the meter running since 1987."[37]

Conclusion

Rivers was different from most comedians. She was funny and very quick with her humor. Her jokes spewed from her mouth like water rushing from a tap, flowing in a quick stream of consciousness with no end in sight. She often asked her audience, "Can we talk?"—a Jewish expression she wove into her act.[38] It soon became her trademark.

One can't help marvel at Rivers's wit and self-deprecating humor. "Never be afraid to laugh at yourself," she once said.[38] "After all, you could be missing out on the joke of the century."[38]

Despite her advice to women to ignore aging, Rivers was also famous for her many cosmetic surgeries.[38] "With all the plastic surgery I've had," she posted on Twitter in 2010, "I'm worried that when I die, God won't recognize me!"[38]

There's no doubt Rivers's feud with Carson left an indelible mark on her psyche. She talked about it all the time. "I adored Johnny," she told the *Hollywood Reporter*.[39] "The Carson breakup hurt me a lot."[39]

In 2015, Verne Gay of *Newsday* tried to settle the matter of who was right, Carson or Rivers.[40] He concluded they were both to blame. Yes, Rivers should have consulted with Carson before she made her decision to sign with Fox, but Carson was also wrong. He should have known NBC had no intention of handing over *The Tonight Show* to a woman.[40] It was a different time back then.

The rift between Rivers and Carson didn't end until he died. While Carson never reconciled with Rivers, Rivers expressed her apology twenty-two years after their feud began.[41] "I loved him so much. It just hurts to lose a friend and not to make amends," she said, as she stood by Carson's memorial grave in Los Angeles, tears streaming down her face. "If I hurt you, I'm sorry. But you hurt me too. Wherever you are, I really miss you, and I thank you."[41] It was better late than never, but it wasn't the same as if they had resolved their differences while Carson was still alive.

Rivers's death from therapeutic complications following a routine, outpatient procedure was devastating, both to her family and to her fans.[42] "At my funeral, I want Meryl Streep crying in five different accents," Rivers once said.[43] She left us laughing to the end.

CHAPTER 22

Prince

Died April 21, 2016

PRINCE, A TALENTED musician whose favorite color was purple, had undergone hip replacement surgery in 2006, but he continued to have significant pain.[1] According to Mark Metz, an attorney for Carver County Sheriff's Office, Prince had been treating himself with pain medications for many years despite there being no known records of any prescriptions for painkillers in his name.[1]

On April 7, 2016, Prince was seen by Dr. Michael Schulenberg of the North Memorial Clinic in Minnetonka, Minnesota, complaining he had vomited the previous night and had numbness and tingling in his hands and legs.[2] Schulenberg administered Prince an intravenous infusion of saline solution, a physiologically compatible solution of salt water, and gave him a prescription for vitamin D and another for an antinausea medication.[2] In keeping with Prince's interest in maintaining his privacy, the doctor wrote the two prescriptions in Kirk Johnson's name, Prince's assistant.[3]

Johnson contacted Schulenberg on April 14 to let him know Prince was having hip pain and needed something to treat his pain before leaving for Atlanta.[4] Having already examined Prince a week earlier, Schulenberg prescribed fifteen Percocet pills, a combination of oxycodone, an opioid drug, and acetaminophen, an over-the-counter pain reliever.[4] As before, he wrote the prescription in Johnson's name.[4] Later that day, Prince flew in his private plane to Atlanta, where he performed two shows.[5] According to the Atlanta promoter, Prince thought his performances were "the best ever."[5]

After the second show, Prince flew back to Minnesota, but just over an hour into the flight, the pilot radioed the control tower to say he had a medical emergency aboard the plane.[6] The plane was diverted to Moline, Illinois, where emergency responders were waiting on the tarmac. [7] Prince, who was unconscious, was resuscitated with two doses of naloxone, an antidote for an opioid overdose, after which he was taken to an area hospital.[7] But despite medical advice to the contrary, he was released after just a few hours and flown to Paisley Park, his compound in Chanhassen, Minnesota.[7] This may have been the first time Prince's closest friends became aware he was addicted to painkillers.

Concerned about Prince's opioid use, Johnson contacted Schulenberg on April 18.[8] Two days later, the physician again examined Prince, but this time, he not only administered intravenous fluids, he also took blood and wrote a prescription for clonidine, a drug that lowers blood pressure and relieves symptoms of opioid withdrawal, and a second prescription for an antihistamine.[8] After he saw the doctor, Prince returned to his private estate.[9]

That evening, Schulenberg contacted Johnson and urged him to have Prince admitted to a chemical dependency treatment progam.[10] Someone on Prince's management team immediately contacted Dr. Howard Kornfeld, founder and medical director of Recovery without Walls, a treatment center in Mill Valley, California, for people addicted to pain medication.[11] Kornfeld was unable to go to Chanhassen, but he sent his son, Andrew, who was only a premed student, on an overnight flight in his place.[11] Andrew was to arrive at Paisley Park sometime in the morning to meet with

Prince and to outline the treatment plan for his recovery, but tragically, Prince died before the meeting could take place.[11]

On the morning of April 21, Johnson tried to contact Prince, but he couldn't reach him.[12] A search of Paisley Park was initiated, and at 9:43 a.m., Prince was found alone in an elevator.[13] Unresponsive, he appeared to have been dead for at least six hours.[14] Schulenberg had planned to take the results of the blood tests to Paisley Park sometime that morning, but by the time he arrived, paramedics were already there.

Prince was pronounced dead at 10:07 a.m.[15] He was fifty-seven years old. Prophetically, five days before he died, he hosted a party for about three hundred guests and told the crowd, "Wait a few days before you waste your prayers."[16] They all assumed he was referring to his medical emergency aboard the plane.[17] But was he? Did Prince know something his guests didn't?

The Autopsy

Police determined that Prince's death was neither a homicide nor a suicide, as the body had no obvious signs of injury or trauma.[18]

A press release provided by the Midwest Medical Examiner's Office of Carver County noted that Prince was five feet three inches tall and weighed 112 pounds.[19] Also, a scar was identified on Prince's left hip, probably from a hip replacement surgery, and another on the lower part of his right leg.[19]

Toxicology analysis detected fentanyl, an opioid, in Prince's blood, the concentration of which was sixty-eight times more than the average amount previously reported in people who had died from a fentanyl overdose. [20] In addition, a potentially lethal amount of fentanyl was found in Prince's stomach, suggesting he took the drug orally.[20]

Fentanyl is a synthetic opioid drug that is one hundred times more potent than morphine and thirty to fifty times more potent than heroin.[21] Like heroin, death from a fentanyl overdose is caused by severe respiratory depression.[21] According to the Centers for Disease Control and Prevention, fentanyl is frequently mixed with heroin, cocaine, or both when sold illegally. [21] However, there was no evidence that either heroin or cocaine or any of their metabolites was present in Prince's blood.[21]

Cause and Manner of Death

Two years after Prince died, Metz, the attorney for Carver County Sheriff's Office, announced that Prince's death was an accident caused by fentanyl toxicity from a self-administered fentanyl overdose.[22] Percocet, the drug Schulenberg had prescribed, was not implicated in Prince's death.[23]

Life and Career

Born in Minneapolis, Minnesota, Prince taught himself to play the piano, guitar, and drums at a very young age.[24] When he was twelve, he already knew he wanted a career in music.[24] In high school, Prince and two of his friends formed a band called Grand Central.[25] At seventeen, he contributed guitar tracks for the band 94 East.[26]

Prince signed his first record deal with Warner Brothers in 1976, after he was introduced to Owen Husney, who helped him create a demo record.[26] "Even at that young age, he was very focused, very directed and highly intelligent," Husney said.[26] "He was creating a whole new sound—the 'Minneapolis Sound.'"[26] When Prince expressed an interest to produce his own record, the studio balked.[27] However, they eventually relented, making the nineteen-year-old Prince the youngest producer ever associated with the record company.[27]

Prince's 1978 album, *For You*, was followed in 1979 by *Prince*.[27] It contained two songs that did especially well—"Why You Wanna Treat Me So Bad?" and "I Wanna Be Your Lover."[27] His album *Dirty Mind*, a "stunning, audacious amalgam of funk, new wave, R&B and pop," was so sexually explicit that, according to Stephen Erlewine, "Prince left nothing to hide."[28]

In 1982, Prince released his album *1999*.[29] It was followed two years later by his classic album, *Purple Rain*.[29] The music from *Purple Rain* served as the soundtrack for the film of the same name.[29] It won an Academy Award for Best Original Song Score that year.[29] Other albums followed, including *Around the World in a Day* (1985), *Parade* (1986), *Sign o' the Times* (1987), *Lovesexy* (1988), and the soundtrack to *Batman* (1989).[29]

Prince's new band, New Power Generation, was launched in the 1990s, but sales of its album, *Love Symbol*, were not spectacular. This caused friction between Prince and Warner Brothers, and as a result, Prince severed ties with his record label and changed his name to an esoteric and unpronounceable fusion of male and female astrological symbols.[29] The media was unable to say Prince's new name, so it referred to him instead as "The Artist Formerly Known as Prince."[29] In 2000, he changed his name back to Prince.[29]

In 2004, Prince won two Grammys for his album *Musicology*.[29] In the same year, he was inducted into the Rock and Roll Hall of Fame.[29] In 2006, he won a Golden

Globe Award for Best Original Song for the score in the animated film *Happy Feet*.[29] Billboard.com proclaimed Prince "the greatest Super Bowl performer ever" after he performed in the 2007 Super Bowl XLI halftime show.[29] He continued to appear in live concerts and to release several albums until he died in 2016.[29]

If there is one thing that can be said about Prince, the multitalented singer, songwriter, and performer, it is that he was a very spiritual and intensely private person. He didn't have a cell phone and rarely gave interviews. However, when he did, as when he appeared on *Larry King Live* on December 10, 1999, he was eloquent, insightful, and candid.[30] "I think my music is inspirational," he told King. "My inspiration comes from God."[30]

Time magazine named Prince "one of the one hundred most influential people in the world" in 2010.[31] Upon hearing of Prince's death, Elton John described him as "the best live performer" he had ever seen.[31]

Paisley Park, Prince's home and studio, was officially opened to the public in October 2016.[32] A month later, Prince's song "Moonbeam Levels" was released posthumously.[32]

In 2019, Prince's memoir, *The Beautiful Ones*, was finally published.[33] It was named "one of the best music books of the year" by the *New York Times* book review and the *Washington Post*.[33]

Conclusion

The Drug Enforcement Administration, or DEA, had been concerned about the dangers of fentanyl ever since fentanyl shipments were seized in northeastern United States and California.[34] Deaths related to fentanyl have been rising in Minnesota since 2000, so when it was determined that Prince died from a fentanyl overdose, the Carver County Sheriff's Office, in association with the DEA, immediately began an investigation.[35]

A large number of pill bottles containing different pharmaceuticals, including Vicodin, a combination of hydrocodone, an opioid drug, and the nonnarcotic pain reliever, acetaminophen, were found at Paisley Park, but none of the medications had been prescribed to Prince.[36] Many pills were not in their original pharmacy-dispensed containers.[37] More than sixty pills were inside a Bayer aspirin bottle, twenty more were inside an Aleve bottle, and a loose pill was found in Prince's bed.[37] Ten of the fifteen Percocet tablets prescribed by Schulenberg were discovered inside Prince's suitcase.[37]

Numerous capsule-shaped tablets branded "Watson 853" were located at Paisley Park, including fifteen in Prince's dressing room.[37] Watson 853-branded pills are a generic form of Vicodin manufactured by Watson Pharmaceuticals.[37] However, when some of the caplets were analyzed, they were found to contain fentanyl instead of Vicodin.[37]

Investigators found no evidence Prince or anybody in his management team knew the counterfeit pills contained fentanyl.[37] In all likelihood, Prince thought he was swallowing Vicodin pills when he was taking the counterfeit medication.[37]

Synthetic opioids were involved in 50 percent of all opioid-related deaths in the United States in 2016, the year Prince died, up from 14 percent in 2010.[38] Most of the deaths were from illegal, counterfeit versions of fentanyl.[38] Because fentanyl is cheap to produce, it is often smuggled into the United States and pressed or encapsulated into pricier, counterfeit prescription pain drugs.[39] Sadly, Vicodin, the drug Prince ingested, was one of those counterfeit pills.

After a two-year investigation into Prince's death, Metz announced in a news conference on April 19, 2018, "There is no reliable evidence showing how Prince obtained the counterfeit Vicodin laced with fentanyl or who else may have had a role in delivering the counterfeit Vicodin to Prince. Without probable cause and no identified suspect, the Carver County Attorney's Office cannot file any criminal charges involving the death of Prince."[40]

Although Schulenberg was not responsible for Prince's death, in trying to help him with his pain, he was held accountable for writing a prescription for Percocet, a controlled substance, in Johnson's name, knowing the medication was actually meant for Prince.[41] On April 26, 2018, the United States Attorney's Office agreed to a civil settlement, the terms of which included a $30,000 fine and monitoring for two years by the DEA.[41] However, Schulenberg's DEA registration was not revoked, thereby permitting him to continue to practice medicine and to prescribe opioids.[41]

CHAPTER 23

Carrie Fisher

Died December 27, 2016

ON DECEMBER 23, 2016, Carrie Fisher, an actress best known for her portrayal of Princess Leia in *Star Wars,* was returning to Los Angeles after taping an episode in London for the Amazon series *Catastrophe.*[1] Sleeping next to her personal assistant during the eleven-hour flight, Fisher had multiple episodes of sleep apnea, periods when she would stop breathing that could last up to ten seconds.[2] This was normal for her.

Fisher had been suffering from sleep apnea for many years, an affliction of which the public was unaware. But approximately twenty minutes before the plane was to land, she vomited profusely, slumped over, became unresponsive, and couldn't be aroused.[3] CPR was initiated by other passengers, and the pilot alerted the airport of the medical emergency aboard the plane. By the time they landed in California, Fisher had stabilized to a normal pulse, but her blood pressure continued to fluctuate.[4] She was rushed to Ronald Reagan UCLA Hospital, where her blood pressure returned to normal, but her pupils were dilated, most likely because there was a period in which she lost oxygen to her eyes and brain.[4]

For a time, there was confusion about the type of medical emergency Fisher had experienced aboard the plane.[5] The early press reports said she had suffered a massive heart attack, a condition in which some of the heart muscle dies, but the first responders labeled her episode a cardiac arrest, as when the heart stops beating entirely due to a defect in the heart's electrical conduction.[6] The hospital, however, found no evidence of a heart attack, and an echocardiogram showed Fisher's heart was pumping normally.[7] Although Fisher underwent dialysis, she never regained consciousness.[8]

Two days after Christmas, Fisher went into cardiac arrest.[9] She was pronounced dead at 8:55 a.m. Her untimely death was a shock to everyone who knew her and to all her fans.

The Autopsy

An autopsy must be performed when there is suspicion of foul play or of an infectious or contagious disease, as well as in the deaths of infants and inmates. If these guidelines are not met, it is at the discretion of the coroner with the approval of the family whether an autopsy should be performed.[10] In Fisher's case, the family didn't grant Dr. Rogers, now the acting chief medical examiner-coroner of the county of Los Angeles, permission to conduct an autopsy.[11] This significantly impaired his ability to gather the relevant information he would need to formulate an informed opinion about the likely cause of Fisher's death. Instead, he had to rely on a whole body CT scan to view the internal organs.[12] As for the toxicology tests, Rogers had to depend on blood and urine collected at the hospital four days before Fisher died.[13] It was far from ideal.

An external examination of Fisher's body failed to yield anything remarkable except for dental implants and a tattoo of a moon and stars on the right ankle.[14] A CT scan of the head revealed no skull fractures or a brain hemorrhage, only mild brain atrophy consistent with Fisher's age. However, a scan of the heart identified mild enlargement with mild calcification in the coronary arteries, not significant enough to have caused a heart attack.[14] Also, moderate to severe arthritic changes were apparent throughout the spine.

In the absence of anatomical changes that could help explain why Fisher died, I then looked to the toxicology report to provide the necessary information. Unfortunately, because Fisher's blood was collected at the hospital four days prior to her death, interpreting the results would prove to be difficult. Hampering the analysis further was the lack of sufficient blood to conduct many of the tests.[14]

Cause and Manner of Death

A toxicology screen of Fisher's hospital-obtained blood, which was subject to false positive results, identified the presence of Ecstasy, methadone, and "other opioids." [14] Most likely, the other opioids was morphine, a major metabolite of heroin, since a second heroin metabolite was found in the vitreous humor, the gel-like substance between the lens and the retina of the eye.[14] The blood also contained a cocaine metabolite, but since there wasn't enough blood, it was impossible to test for the presence of free, unmetabolized cocaine.[14] Without the ability to quantify the concentration of any of the drugs detected in Fisher's system, their contribution to her death couldn't be determined.

Cocaethylene, a substance synthesized by the liver from cocaine and alcohol, wasn't found in Fisher's blood, as neither was alcohol, although alcohol was present in the urine.[15] However, the presence of a cocaine metabolite in Fisher's blood and alcohol in her urine meant that Fisher must have consumed cocaine and alcohol sometime before her medical emergency. Most likely, the two drugs weren't taken at the same time since cocaethylene wasn't detected in Fisher's blood. Also, by the time Fisher experienced her medical emergency, alcohol was already being excreted from her body.

Low, therapeutic levels of fluoxetine, an antidepressant medication, and meperidine, an opioid drug, as well as diphenhydramine, an antihistamine, were identified in Fisher's liver. However, the contribution of these drugs to Fisher's death couldn't be evaluated.

Rogers was aware that Fisher's heart had stopped beating and that she had experienced several episodes of sleep apnea while on the plane. He also knew that several opioid drugs that cause respiratory depression were detected in her blood. His frustration was clearly apparent in his writing of the autopsy report.
[16] "Based on the available toxicological information, limited history of present illness [and the] lack of correlating symptoms and medical observation, there are significant limitations in one's ability to interpret the toxicology results and their contribution to cause of

death," Rogers wrote in the autopsy report.[16] Unable to link any drug present in Fisher's system to her death, Rogers labeled the cause of death as sleep apnea but added the phrase, "and other undetermined factors," specifically mentioning drug use and atherosclerotic heart disease as contributing factors.[16]

It would have been simpler for Rogers to label the cause of Fisher's death as "cardiac arrest" or "respiratory arrest," but it wouldn't have been within the guidelines prescribed in the *Physicians' Handbook on Medical Certification of Death*.[17] The handbook clearly states, "The immediate cause does not mean the mechanism of death or terminal event as, for example, cardiac arrest or respiratory arrest," and these examples "should not be reported as the immediate cause of death as they are a statement not specifically related to the disease process."[17]

As for the manner of death, Rogers labeled it "undetermined" because the limited information provided in the autopsy and toxicology tests couldn't exclude any one of the other four categories—natural, suicide, homicide, or accidental.[18] Under the circumstances, it was the best he could have done.

Life and Career

Fisher was born in 1956 to Debbie Reynolds, a Protestant actress who was known as "America's Sweetheart," and Eddie Fisher, a twenty-seven-year-old Jewish crooner who, with his strong and infectious tenor voice, was one of the most popular singers of his time.[19] Reynolds divorced Eddie Fisher in 1959 when she discovered he had been having an affair with Elizabeth Taylor, the twenty-six-year-old widow of their best friend, Mike Todd, once voted "the most beautiful woman in the world."[20] In *Wishful Drinking*, her one-woman show, Fisher would recount how her father "rushed to Elizabeth Taylor's side and gradually moved to her front."[21] The bad publicity caused by Eddie Fisher's divorce forced NBC to cancel his popular television show, whereas Reynolds, as the "wronged wife," came out of the ordeal unscathed.[22] Reynolds remarried when Fisher was four years old.[22] Her new husband was Harry Karl, a Jewish shoe magnate.[22]

Fisher always claimed she was an enthusiastic agnostic. However, with her father and stepfather both Jewish, she was exposed to Jewish customs and traditions for nearly all her formative years. As an adult, she occasionally attended Jewish services with her orthodox Jewish friends and was briefly married to a Jewish singer-songwriter, Paul Simon.[23] "I always felt the Jewish part more," Fisher said about being the daughter of a Protestant mother and a Jewish father.[23] "In fact, growing up I felt like a Jew among WASPs."[23] This may help explain why the family refused to give permission for an autopsy to be done when Fisher died. With few exceptions, autopsies are not permitted in the Jewish religion. Of course, it's also possible the family simply didn't want to know what caused Fisher's death.

When she was seventeen years old, Fisher made her stage debut as a singer in the hit Broadway show *Irene*.[23] Two years later, she appeared alongside Warren Beatty, Julie Christie, and Goldie Hawn in the film *Shampoo*.[23]

On May 25, 1977, the public was introduced to Fisher as Princess Leia in the science fiction space opera *Star Wars*.[24] Along with her costars—Mark Hamill as Luke Skywalker, Harrison Ford as Han Solo, Alex Guinness as Obi-Wan Kenobi, and the loveable robot, R2-D2—Fisher helped the Rebel Alliance prevent the galaxy from being destroyed by the mysterious and cruel Darth Vader.[24] Two weeks after the film's debut, people were talking about Princess Leia and "the bar scene"—set in a dimly lit cantina frequented by assorted strange and exotic alien characters.[25]

Fisher's success in *Star Wars* led to other roles, including in *Hannah and her Sisters* and *When Harry Met Sally*, as well as to several television appearances and a special with Ringo Starr, formerly of the Beatles.[26] However, despite her appearance in other highly popular films, Fisher would always be identified with Princess Leia in *Star Wars* and its sequels, *The Empire Strikes Back* and *Return of the Jedi*.

In her one-woman show, *Wishful Drinking*, Fisher envisioned the way her life would end.[27] "However I go, I want it reported that I drowned in moonlight, strangled by my own bra," she wrote.[27] The reality was quite different. Her death was sudden and unexpected.

Conclusion

It was well known that Fisher had been battling bipolar disorder for many years. She was very open about her diagnosis and even spoke about it in 2004 at the annual meeting of the American Psychiatric Association.[28] Bipolar disorder "took a hold when I was fourteen or fifteen," she said in 2013.[29] The neurological brain disorder causes intense mood swings and changes in energy and activity levels ranging from manic episodes of extremely elated and energized behavior to very sad or hopeless periods described as depressive episodes.[30]

Drugs, such as LSD, and Percodan, a combination of aspirin and the opioid drug, oxycodone, both of which Fisher admitted to taking throughout the 1970s and 1980s, as well as cocaine, which she was taking when she was filming *The Empire Strikes Back* and *Return of the Jedi*, helped Fisher to function and to deal with the effects of her bipolar disorder.[31] "Drugs made me feel normal," Fisher said in a 2001 interview in *Psychology Today*.[32] "They contained me." Unfortunately, she also became addicted and once almost died from a drug overdose.[33] "I couldn't stop, or stay stopped," Fisher told *People* magazine in 1987.[34] "It was never my fantasy to have a drug problem."[34]

In 2016, Harvard College presented Fisher with its Annual Outstanding Lifetime Achievement Award in Cultural Humanism, stating, "Her forthright activism and outspokenness about addiction, mental health and agnosticism have advanced public discourse on these issues with creativity and empathy."[35]

What was not widely reported, and of which Fisher purposely never spoke about publicly, was that she suffered from sleep apnea. Whether it truly was the cause of her death will never be known. Her body was cremated and is no longer available for further testing.

And so, Fisher is now "in a galaxy far, far away." I have no doubt she is well taken care of, and our memories of her and her legacy will long outlive her death. "When I arrived, I was virtually unattended!" Fisher wrote in *The Princess Diarist*.[36] "And I have been trying to make up for that fact ever since. Perpetual celebrity, the kind where any mention of you will interest a significant percentage of the public until the day you die ... is exceedingly rare."[36]

"May the force be with you, Carrie Fisher."

CHAPTER 24

Conclusion

HAVING REVIEWED THE science behind the deaths of famous people, I was saddened to discover that drug use was implicated in 70 percent of the deaths, eleven of which were due to an overdose. Most often, the drugs involved included chloral hydrate, heroin, cocaine, a speedball—a mixture of cocaine and heroin— or polypharmacy, a combination of benzodiazepines, opioids, amphetamines, antihistamines, or alcohol.

Four celebrities were determined to have died from natural causes—Errol Flynn, Cass Elliot, Elvis Presley, and Karen Carpenter. However, an injection of meperidine, an opioid analgesic, may have expedited Flynn's death. All of these deaths could have been prevented with a change in lifestyle, a change in diet, and, in the case of Elliot, possibly surgery.

Two celebrity deaths were the result of suicide— Robin Williams by hanging and Marilyn Monroe from an overdose of chloral hydrate, a sedative. However, while Anna Nicole Smith ingested an overdose of the same drug as Monroe, her death was ruled an accident.

Jimi Hendrix choked on vomit due to an overdose of barbiturates. The manner of his death was undetermined; however, in my opinion, it should have been ruled accidental.

Two homicides were among this group of celebrities. JonBenét Ramsey was strangled, but her perpetrator was never apprehended, while Michael Jackson died after he was medically sedated by his physician with propofol. Jackson's doctor spent two years in prison for breaching the standard of care by administering the anesthetic in a nonhospital setting and without the proper equipment for monitoring and resuscitation.

Jackson's wasn't the only death in which physician error was implicated. Joan Rivers died from "therapeutic complications" while undergoing minor outpatient surgical procedures. Her physicians paid a substantial financial settlement for their negligence.

Two famous people died by drowning—Natalie Wood in the Pacific Ocean and Whitney Houston in a hotel bathtub filled with twelve inches of scalding water. However, while police closed their investigation of Houston's death, they have maintained Wood's file open, now nearly forty years.

Alcohol intoxication was the cause of Amy Winehouse's death. It was also implicated in Natalie Wood's death and was a contributing factor in the onset of fatty metamorphosis in Errol Flynn and Janis Joplin. However, while Elvis Presley suffered from the same condition, in his case, the fatty liver was caused by obesity.

Brittany Murphy's death from multiple drug intoxication was ruled an accident. However, the manner of Carrie Fisher's death was undetermined since her family didn't give permission for an autopsy and toxicology tests to be done.

Forensics revealed that being too thin can be just as deadly as being too heavy. Karen Carpenter and Cass Elliot were both young, thirty-two and thirty-three years old, respectively, and they each had a weight problem. Carpenter's weight was too low, whereas Elliot was significantly overweight. Carpenter and Elliot were both singers and were acutely aware of the importance of body image as they chased fame and glory. Carpenter zealously pursued weight loss with laxatives and thyroid pills. She suffered from anorexia nervosa, an eating disorder, and died from toxic effects to the heart. Elliot died from congestive heart failure caused by her obesity.

Autopsy and postmortem toxicology tests exposed that too much of a good thing isn't good for you either. Prior to his death, Errol Flynn's lifestyle was one of excess—too much alcohol, too many women, and too much spending. However, Flynn paid a heavy price for living in the fast lane, the cost of which was cirrhosis of the liver, coronary atherosclerosis, genital warts, and death at a young age.

In this group of celebrities, drug use was clearly identified as a risk factor for heart disease. Elvis Presley and Whitney Houston, two celebrities who had abused drugs over many years, both suffered from coronary atherosclerosis—plaque in the arteries. Sam Kinison, John Belushi, and Robin Williams, as well as Flynn and Presley, famous people who had a history of abusing alcohol or drugs at some point in their lives, all had an enlarged heart, a risk factor for sudden death from an arrhythmia, an electrical abnormality in the heart.

Neither status, wealth, nor beauty was sufficient to prevent acquiring common human ailments and disorders from which many ordinary people suffer. Like many men in their age group, Michael Jackson and Robin Williams also suffered from an enlarged prostate. In Jackson's case, he also had a benign colon polyp and osteoarthritis. However, famous men weren't the only ones who suffered from everyday afflictions. Whitney Houston had uterine fibroids, Anna Nicole Smith suffered from Hashimoto thyroid disease, and Brittany Murphy was plagued by heavy menstrual bleeding. These autopsy findings confirmed that when it comes to biology and disease, celebrities are not any different from anybody else.

If there is one lesson to be learned from my analysis of the science behind the deaths of famous people, it is that drugs can kill. Nearly half of all the celebrity deaths were from a drug overdose. The question remains, therefore, Why do celebrities use drugs?

Some have suggested that drug use enhances creativity, but there is little scientific basis to support this theory. [1] Others have claimed entertainers use opioids and sedatives to relieve stress and to calm them down after late-night performances. Since many entertainers command exorbitant earnings, and since illicit drugs are readily available in their professional circles, famous people have the means to support a drug habit. However, no matter the reason, once opioid or illegal drugs are consumed, tolerance and drug addiction can develop, leading to incrementally higher drug intake, with death often following from an accidental overdose.

One of the best ways to combat substance abuse is through education. To reduce the number of drug-related fatalities among celebrities, it's important that, just like the general population, famous people should become more fully aware of the risks posed by pharmaceuticals, illicit drugs, and polypharmacy, as well as with the scientific concepts of tolerance and addiction. "Just Say No" to drugs, a slogan proposed by First Lady Nancy Reagan in the late 1980s during the war on drugs, is not only appropriate for children, it is also applicable to adults.

FORMULARY

Acetaminophen (Tylenol)

Acetaminophen is an over-the-counter medication that relieves pain and lowers fever. The drug was discovered by accident in the late nineteenth century. The US Food and Drug Administration, or FDA, first issued a patent for acetaminophen in 1951. Unlike aspirin, acetaminophen doesn't cause stomach ulcers or gastrointestinal upset. However, when taken long-term or in higher than recommended doses, it can damage the liver and may even cause death.

Actifed

Actifed is a combination medication composed of pseudoephedrine, a nasal decongestant, and tripolidine, an antihistamine. The drug is used for the relief of symptoms associated with allergies and the common cold.

Alcohol

Alcohol, also known as ethanol, depresses the central nervous system and can impair judgment, reduce inhibition and reaction time, diminish fine motor control, and cause sedation. Tolerance, physical dependence, and withdrawal symptoms may develop after long-term use. The blood alcohol concentration, or BAC, legal limit for drivers in the United States is eighty milligrams per deciliter.

Alprazolam (Xanax)

Alprazolam is an antianxiety medication of the benzodiazepine class of pharmaceuticals. The drug was first introduced to the United States market in 1981. Alprazolam facilitates the action of gamma aminobutyric acid, an inhibitory biochemical neurotransmitter in the brain. The FDA specifically warns against the simultaneous use of benzodiazepine and opioid drugs, the combination of which can cause profound sedation, respiratory depression, coma, and death.

Amoxicillin

Amoxicillin is a penicillin antibiotic medication that kills certain types of bacteria. It is one of the most commonly prescribed antibiotic medicines in children. The drug interferes with the synthesis of the bacterial cell wall, allowing for leakage of the cellular contents and leading to death of the bacteria.

D-Amphetamine

D-Amphetamine is one of the most potent drugs that stimulate the central nervous system. It causes wakefulness, alertness, a decreased sense of fatigue, mood elevation, an ability to concentrate, as well as elation and euphoria. When taken in large doses over an extended duration, the stimulating effect of D-amphetamine is almost always followed by depression and fatigue.

Aspirin

Aspirin is an over-the-counter medication that relieves pain and lowers fever. When taken long-term, it may cause gastrointestinal upset and ringing in the ears. The drug's popularity declined in 1956 after the development of acetaminophen and further declined in 1962 after the introduction of ibuprofen.

Atropine

Atropine blocks the action of acetylcholine, a biochemical neurotransmitter at nerve endings in smooth muscle, secretory glands, and the central nervous system. The drug increases cardiac output, dries mucus secretions, and is an antidote for several pesticides. Atropine is well absorbed, and its action lasts three to four hours.

Barbiturate

Barbiturate is a class of pharmaceuticals that depress the central nervous system. Drugs in this class produce a wide range of effects, including sedation. Most barbiturate overdoses involve a combination of barbiturates with other central nervous system depressant drugs, such as alcohol or opiates.

Benzodiazepine

Benzodiazepine is a class of psychoactive pharmaceutical drugs used to treat anxiety or as sedatives. The FDA specifically warns against the simultaneous use of benzodiazepine and opioid drugs, the combination of which can cause profound sedation, respiratory depression, coma, and death.

Butabarbital

Butabarbital is a barbiturate drug that depresses the central nervous system. It is used to treat insomnia or as a sedative before surgery. Most barbiturate overdoses involve a combination of a barbiturate drug with other central nervous system depressant drugs, including alcohol and opiates.

Caffeine

Caffeine is a drug with mild central nervous system stimulant properties. It is present in over-the-counter cold preparations, some foods and drinks, and is often added to pain relievers and products that keep a person alert. When taken in high doses, caffeine can cause restlessness, insomnia, a rapid heart rhythm, and anxiety.

Cascara

Cascara is a laxative that causes the muscles of the bowels to contract, thereby helping to move the stool through the bowels.

Chloral Hydrate

Chloral hydrate is a central nervous system depressant drug that is rapidly metabolized to trichloroethanol, which is largely responsible for the sedative and hypnotic properties of chloral hydrate. When taken in an overdose, chloral hydrate can cause respiratory depression, coma, arrhythmia, and death. In 2012, chloral hydrate was taken off the market due to oversedation in children and possible liver damage upon long-term use.

Chlordiazepoxide (Librium)

Chlordiazepoxide is a sedative and hypnotic drug of the benzodiazepine class of pharmaceuticals. The drug was the first benzodiazepine medication to be synthesized and was marketed in the United States in 1960. Chlordiazepoxide is used to treat anxiety, insomnia, and alcohol withdrawal symptoms. It is believed to enhance the activity of gamma aminobutyric acid, the major inhibitory biochemical neurotransmitter in the brain. The FDA specifically warns against the simultaneous use of benzodiazepine and opioid drugs, the combination of which can cause profound sedation, respiratory depression, coma, and death.

Chlorpheniramine

Chlorpheniramine reduces the symptoms of the common cold or hay fever, including sneezing, itching, watery eyes, and runny nose caused by histamine, a natural biochemical in the body. Due to the mild sedative properties of chlorpheniramine, caution is advised when taking the drug with other central nervous system depressants.

Ciprofloxacin (Cipro)

Ciprofloxacin is an antibiotic medication used to treat skin, bone, joint, respiratory, sinus, and urinary tract infections, as well as certain cases of diarrhea. The drug was first introduced to the United States in 1987. It is on the World Health Organization's List of Essential Medicines, the safest and most effective medicines needed in a health system. Some of the more serious side effects of ciprofloxacin include tendon problems, nerve damage, and mood or behavioral changes.

Clarithromycin (Biaxin)

Clarithromycin was invented in 1980 by researchers at the Japanese drug company Taisho Pharmaceutical. This antibiotic medication is used to treat bacterial infections affecting the skin and respiratory system. It can also be used with other medicines to treat stomach ulcers.

Clonazepam (Klonapin)

Clonazepam is an antiseizure and antipanic drug in the benzodiazepine class of pharmaceuticals. It is believed to enhance the activity of gamma aminobutyric acid, the major inhibitory biochemical neurotransmitter in the brain. The FDA specifically warns against the simultaneous use of benzodiazepine and opioid drugs, the combination of which can cause profound sedation, respiratory depression, coma, and death.

Clonidine

Clonidine is an antihypertensive drug used to treat high blood pressure. It lowers blood pressure by changing nerve impulses in the brain, so blood vessels relax and blood passes through the vessels more easily.

Cocaine

Cocaine is a powerfully addictive drug that stimulates the central nervous system and increases the levels of dopamine, a biochemical neurotransmitter in the brain. Cocaine causes mental alertness, hypersensitivity to sight, sound, and touch, as well as irritability and paranoia. The effects of cocaine appear almost immediately and disappear within a few minutes to an hour, depending on whether it is injected, smoked, or snorted. Some of the most severe side effects of a cocaine overdose include arrhythmia, a heart attack, stroke, difficulty breathing, high blood pressure, hallucinations, and extreme agitation or anxiety. There is no specific antidote to reverse a cocaine overdose.

Codeine

Codeine is an opioid drug that is seven to fourteen times less potent than morphine. It is used to treat cough and to relieve mild to moderately severe pain. Some side effects of codeine include sedation, mental clouding, euphoria, agitation, abdominal bloating, nausea, vomiting, and constipation. When taken in higher than therapeutic doses, codeine is less likely to cause respiratory depression than morphine. However, when combined with other central nervous system depressant drugs, especially at higher doses, codeine can cause respiratory distress and death.

Cyclizine

Cyclizine is an antinausea medication that prevents vomiting and dizziness caused by motion sickness.

Cyclobenzaprine (Flexeril)

Cyclobenzaprine is a muscle relaxant medication that, along with rest and physical therapy, is used to relieve muscle spasm and muscle pain of local origin. It is ineffective in relieving muscle spasm, injury, or pain caused by central nervous system disease.

Dexamethasone

Dexamethasone is a corticosteroid drug that decreases inflammation. Long-term use of large doses of dexamethasone can lead to changes in body fat, increased acne or facial hair, menstrual problems, and erectile dysfunction. When taken in an overdose, dexamethasone is not expected to be life-threatening.

Dextropropoxyphene (Darvon)

Dextropropoxyphene is an opioid drug that depresses the central nervous system and relieves pain. As with all opioids, the drug can cause respiratory depression and a drop in blood pressure, especially when taken in larger than therapeutic doses. In 2010, dextropropoxyphene was taken off the market due to numerous cases of accidental or intentional overdoses and for causing serious toxic effects to the heart, even at therapeutic doses.

Diazepam (Valium)

Diazepam is a drug in the benzodiazepine class of pharmaceuticals. It is used to treat various anxiety disorders and to alleviate the symptoms of alcohol withdrawal. Diazepam facilitates the action of gamma aminobutyric acid, an inhibitory biochemical neurotransmitter in the brain. The FDA specifically warns against the simultaneous use of benzodiazepine and opioid drugs, the combination of which can cause profound sedation, respiratory depression, coma, and death.

Diphenhydramine (Benadryl)

Diphenhydramine is an antihistamine medication that reduces the symptoms of the common cold or hay fever, including sneezing, itching, watery eyes, and runny nose caused by histamine, a natural biochemical in the body. Because of its mild sedative properties, caution is advised when taking diphenhydramine with other central nervous system depressant drugs.

Doxylamine

Doxylamine is an antihistamine medication that reduces the symptoms of the common cold or hay fever, including sneezing, itching, watery eyes, and runny nose caused by histamine, a natural biochemical in the body. Because of its mild sedative properties, caution is advised when taking doxylamine with other central nervous system depressant drugs.

Ecstasy

Ecstasy is a drug that produces altered mood and feelings of increased energy, pleasure, emotional warmth, and a distorted perception of sensory input and time. It acts by increasing the activity of three chemicals in the brain—dopamine, norepinephrine, and serotonin. The effects of Ecstasy last about three to six hours. When taken in high doses, Ecstasy can cause liver failure, kidney failure, heart failure, and even death.

Ephedrine

Ephedrine is a decongestant and bronchodilator medication used for the temporary relief of shortness of breath, chest tightness, and wheezing due to bronchial asthma. The drug reduces swelling, constricts blood vessels in the nasal passages, and widens the lung airways for easier breathing.

Escitalopram (Lexapro)

Escitalopram is an antidepressant drug used to treat anxiety in adults and major depressive disorder in adults and adolescents. It affects chemicals in the brain that may be unbalanced in people with depression or anxiety. Escitalopram selectively inhibits the reuptake of serotonin, a biochemical neurotransmitter in the brain, with little to no effect on the reuptake of two other chemicals, norepinephrine and dopamine.

Ethchlorvynol (Placidyl)

Ethchlorvynol is a hypnotic and sedative drug that was popular in the 1950s for the treatment of insomnia. It has since been replaced by more effective medications.

Ethinamate (Valmid)

Ethinamate is a short-acting sedative-hypnotic drug used to treat insomnia. It has been replaced by other more effective sedative-hypnotic medications.

Fentanyl

Fentanyl is a powerful opioid drug that is fifty to one hundred times more potent than morphine. The drug is typically used to treat severe pain and to manage pain after surgery. Fentanyl is sometimes used to treat patients with chronic pain who exhibit tolerance to other opioids. Like with all opioids, when taken in an overdose, fentanyl slows or stops the breathing process, thereby decreasing the amount of oxygen reaching the brain. Coma, permanent brain damage, and death may follow.

Finasteride (Proscar)

Finasteride is used to treat symptoms associated with benign prostatic hyperplasia, commonly known as an enlarged prostate. The FDA approved the drug for human use in 1992. Finasteride reduces the size of the prostate by preventing the conversion of testosterone to dihydrotestosterone.

Fluoxetine (Prozac)

Fluoxetine is an antidepressant medication that affects biochemical neurotransmitters in the brain in people with depression, panic, anxiety, or obsessive-compulsive symptoms. The drug selectively inhibits the reuptake of serotonin with little to no effect on the reuptake of two other chemicals, norepinephrine and dopamine.

Guaifenesin (Mucinex)

Guaifenesin is an over-the-counter expectorant that helps loosen phlegm and mucus in the chest and throat caused by the common cold, infections, and allergies. The drug helps thin bronchial secretions and make coughs more productive.

Heroin

Heroin is a highly addictive opioid drug that depresses the central nervous system. It is two to five times more potent than morphine. Heroin is rapidly metabolized to morphine, which binds to areas of the brain responsible for controlling pain, pleasure, heart rate, sleep, and respiration. When taken in an overdose, heroin slows or stops the breathing process, thereby decreasing the amount of oxygen reaching the brain. Coma, permanent brain damage, and death may follow. Naloxone is a specific antidote to reverse a heroin overdose.

Hydrocodone

Hydrocodone is an opioid drug that is equal in analgesic potency to morphine. As with all opioids, when taken in an overdose, hydrocodone can cause a severe drop in blood pressure. Death from respiratory depression may follow. Naloxone is a specific antidote for a hydrocodone overdose.

Hydroquinone

Used as a topical ointment, hydroquinone decreases the formation of melanin and lightens areas of the skin in vitiligo, freckles, age spots, sun-damaged skin, and darkened skin caused by hormonal changes. The drug produces depigmentation by suppressing metabolic processes of melanocytes in the skin. However, exposure to sunlight will reverse the drug's action and cause repigmentation.

Ibuprofen

Ibuprofen is an over-the-counter nonsteroidal anti-inflammatory medication used to reduce fever and to treat pain or inflammation caused by headache, toothache, back pain, arthritis, menstrual cramps, and minor injury. The FDA specifically warns of an increased risk of serious and potentially fatal cardiovascular thrombotic events, including fatal heart attacks and stroke, from the use of nonsteroidal anti-inflammatory drugs. The risk, which can occur early during treatment, increases with duration.

Ipecac

Ipecac, whose main active ingredient is emetine, is taken by mouth to induce vomiting after suspected poisoning. Vomiting occurs within fifteen to sixty minutes by an irritant action on the bowels.

Ketamine

Ketamine is an oral anesthetic drug that can cause distortion of colors, sounds, self, and one's environment. Because of its hallucinogenic properties, ketamine is sometimes abused and taken as a recreational drug.

Levodopa

Levodopa is a medication used to treat symptoms of Parkinson's disease. The drug is a precursor to dopamine, a biochemical neurotransmitter in the brain.

Lidocaine

Lidocaine is a topical local anesthetic medication used to reduce pain or discomfort caused by skin irritation.

Lorazepam (Ativan)

Lorazepam is an antianxiety drug of the benzodiazepine class of pharmaceuticals. It facilitates the action of gamma aminobutyric acid, an inhibitory biochemical neurotransmitter in the brain. When administered intravenously or intramuscularly, lorazepam produces mild sedation and reduces anxiety prior to surgery. The FDA specifically warns against the simultaneous use of benzodiazepine and opioid drugs, the combination of which may cause profound sedation, respiratory depression, coma, and death.

Lysergic Acid Diethylamide (LSD)

Lysergic acid diethylamide is a hallucinogenic drug whose effects include altered thoughts, feelings, and awareness of one's surroundings. It is illegal in the United States.

Marijuana

Marijuana contains the chemical delta-9-tetrahydrocannabinol, or THC, which is responsible for the psychoactive mind-altering state produced by marijuana. THC alters normal brain communication, especially in areas of the brain that influence pleasure, memory, thinking, concentration, movement, coordination, sensory and time perception. The effects of marijuana begin almost immediately, but they only last one to three hours. However, THC can be detected in the body for days or even weeks after first use. When taken in large doses, marijuana can cause acute psychosis, including hallucinations, delusions, and a loss of a sense of personal identity.

Meperidine (Demerol)

Meperidine is an opioid drug that depresses the central nervous system. It is seven to ten times less potent than morphine. Meperidine is used to treat moderate to severe pain. As with all opioid drugs, when taken as an overdose, meperidine can cause a severe drop in blood pressure. Death may follow from respiratory depression. Naloxone is a specific antidote for a meperidine overdose.

Methadone

Methadone is an opioid drug that depresses the central nervous system. It is three times more potent than morphine. The drug relieves pain and is used as part of a drug addiction detoxification and maintenance program to reduce withdrawal symptoms in people addicted to heroin. As with all opioid drugs, methadone binds to areas of the brain responsible for controlling pain, pleasure, heart rate, sleep, and respiration.

L-Methamphetamine

L-Methamphetamine is the active ingredient in some over-the-counter nasal decongestant inhalers. The drug acts as a vasoconstrictor. Unlike D-methamphetamine, the structural mirror image of L-methamphetamine, the drug does not possess euphoria or addictive properties.

Methaqualone (Quaalude)

Methaqualone is a sedative-hypnotic drug, similar to barbiturates, that depresses the central nervous system. It was popular as a recreational drug from the 1960s to the 1980s but has been illegal in the United States since then.

Midazolam (Versed)

Midazolam is a drug in the benzodiazepine class of pharmaceuticals. It is used to sedate patients prior to minor surgery, dental work, or other medical procedures. Midazolam facilitates the action of gamma aminobutyric acid, an inhibitory biochemical neurotransmitter in the brain. The FDA specifically warns against the simultaneous use of benzodiazepine and opioid drugs, the combination of which can cause profound sedation, respiratory depression, coma, and death.

Midol

Midol is an over-the-counter medication used for the relief of menstrual cramps and to reduce bloating. The active ingredient in Midol is acetaminophen, a nonnarcotic pain reliever, in combination with a diuretic.

Minocycline

Minocycline is a broad spectrum antibiotic medication of the tetracycline class of pharmaceuticals. The drug is used to treat urinary tract, respiratory, and skin infections, as well as severe acne and other ailments caused by bacteria. Birth control pills may be less effective when taken together with minocycline. Children younger than eight years of age should not take this medication since it can cause permanent yellowing or graying of the teeth.

Mirtazapine

Mirtazapine is a drug used to treat major depressive disorders. It is believed to affect communication between nerve cells in the central nervous system and to restore chemical balance in the brain by increasing the release of two biochemical neurotransmitters, norepinephrine and serotonin.

Monobenzone (Benoquin)

Monobenzone is a mild topical depigmenting medication used to treat vitiligo. The drug, which takes one to four months to act, increases excretion of melanin from melanocytes in the skin. Exposure to sunlight reduces the depigmenting effect of monobenzone.

Morphine

Morphine is an opioid drug that depresses the central nervous system. It is also the active metabolite of heroin. Morphine relieves moderate to severe pain by binding to areas of the brain responsible for controlling pain, pleasure, heart rate, sleep, and respiration. When taken in an overdose, morphine can cause a severe drop in blood pressure. Death from respiratory depression may follow. Naloxone is a specific antidote for a morphine overdose.

Naloxone (Narcan)

Naloxone is a drug used to rapidly reverse an opioid overdose. It acts by competitively binding to opioid receptors.

Nystatin

When taken orally, nystatin is used to treat yeast infections in the mouth and stomach. The drug is ineffective for fungal infections in other parts of the body or on the skin. Nystatin acts by binding to certain molecules in the fungal cell membrane, changing the permeability of the cell wall, thereby allowing for leakage of the cellular contents and leading to death of the fungus.

Oseltamivir (Tamiflu)

Oseltamivir is an antiviral drug used to treat flu symptoms caused by influenza virus types A and B. It is most effective the first two days after flu symptoms appear. Oseltamivir may also prevent influenza in people who have been exposed to the influenza virus but have not yet shown any symptoms of the disease.

Oxazepam

Oxazepam is a drug in the benzodiazepine class of pharmaceuticals. It affects chemicals in the brain in people who suffer from anxiety. The FDA specifically warns against the simultaneous use of benzodiazepine and opioid drugs, the combination of which can cause profound sedation, respiratory depression, coma, and death.

Oxycodone

Oxycodone is an opioid drug that is about 50 percent more potent than morphine. The drug is used to treat moderate to severe pain. When taken in an overdose, oxycodone can cause a severe drop in blood pressure. Death from respiratory depression may follow. Naloxone is a specific antidote for an oxycodone overdose.

Pentobarbital (Nembutal)

Pentobarbital is a barbiturate drug that depresses the central nervous system. It has a rapid onset of effect, and its sedative action lasts three to four hours when given in therapeutic doses. When taken in an overdose, symptoms may include extreme drowsiness, slowed or shallow breathing, weak pulse, rapid heart rate, little or no urination, pinpoint or dilated pupils, and feeling cold. Death from respiratory arrest may follow. Pentobarbital is utilized to initiate and maintain medically induced coma, especially in brain injury, and as a means of lethal injection in humans. Most barbiturate overdoses involve a combination of barbiturates with other central nervous system depressant drugs.

Percocet

Percocet is a combination medication consisting of oxycodone, an opioid analgesic drug, and acetaminophen, a nonnarcotic pain reliever. The drug is used to treat moderate to severe pain and is about 50 percent more potent than morphine. When taken in an overdose, Percocet can cause a severe drop in blood pressure. Death from respiratory depression may follow. Naloxone is a specific antidote for a Percocet overdose.

Percodan

Percodan is a combination medication consisting of oxycodone, an opioid analgesic drug, and aspirin, a nonnarcotic pain reliever. The drug is used to treat moderate to severe pain and is about 50 percent more potent than morphine. When taken in an overdose, Percodan can cause a severe drop in blood pressure. Death from respiratory depression may follow. Naloxone is a specific antidote for a Percodan overdose.

Phencyclidine

Phencyclidine is an illegal drug used for its mind-altering effects. It can cause hallucinations, distorted perceptions of sounds, violent behavior, and severe agitation. As a recreational drug, phencyclidine is typically smoked, but it can be taken orally, snorted, or injected. An overdose of phencyclidine can result in serious, adverse symptoms or even death.

Phenobarbital

Phenobarbital is a barbiturate medication used to treat or prevent seizures. The drug is also used as a sedative. Most barbiturate overdoses involve a combination of barbiturates with other central nervous system depressant drugs.

Prednisone

Prednisone is a corticosteroid drug that suppresses the immune system and prevents the release of substances in the body that cause inflammation. It is used to treat allergic disorders, skin conditions, ulcerative colitis, arthritis, lupus, and psoriasis as well as breathing disorders.

Propofol

Propofol is a general anesthetic drug used to sedate patients for surgery or other medical procedures.

Pseudoephedrine

Pseudoephedrine is a medication used to treat nasal and sinus congestion and to drain fluid from the inner ear. The drug acts by shrinking blood vessels in the nasal passages responsible for nasal congestion.

Quetiapine (Seroquel)

Quetiapine is an antipsychotic drug used to treat schizophrenia and bipolar disorder, as well as major depressive disorders when given along with other antidepressant drugs.

Rabeprazole (Aciphex)

Rabeprazole is a proton-pump inhibitor used to treat heartburn, stomach ulcers, gastroesophageal reflux disease, and esophageal damage. The drug acts by reducing secretions of stomach acids.

Sertraline (Zoloft)

Sertraline is an antidepressant drug that affects chemicals in the brain in people with depression, panic, anxiety, or obsessive-compulsive symptoms. The drug is used to treat depression, obsessive-compulsive disorder, anxiety disorders such as panic disorder and social anxiety disorder, as well as posttraumatic stress disorder and premenstrual dysphoric disorder.

Tamsulosin (Flomax)

Tamsulosin is a drug used to treat symptoms caused by benign prostatic hyperplasia, commonly known as an enlarged prostate. The drug relaxes the muscles in the prostate and the bladder neck, making it easier to urinate.

Temazepam (Restoril)

Temazepam is a drug in the benzodiazepine class of pharmaceuticals. It affects chemicals in the brain in people suffering from insomnia. The FDA specifically warns against the simultaneous use of benzodiazepine and opioid drugs, the combination of which can cause profound sedation, respiratory depression, coma, and death.

Topiramate (Topamax)

Topiramate was approved by the FDA for the treatment of seizures in adults and children. The drug can also be used to prevent migraines in adults and teenagers but not for headaches that have already begun.

Tripolidine

Tripolidine is an over-the-counter antihistamine medication used to treat symptoms associated with allergies. The drug is sometimes combined with other cold medications to relieve flulike symptoms.

Vesparax

Vesparax is a combination medication consisting of two barbiturates, secobarbital and brallobarbital, as well as the antihistamine drug hydroxyzine. The medication was used as a sedative but has been replaced by other more effective drugs.

Vicodin

Vicodin is a combination medication consisting of hydrocodone, an opioid analgesic drug, and acetaminophen, a nonnarcotic pain reliever. It is used to treat moderate to moderately severe pain and is similar in potency to morphine. When taken in an overdose, Vicodin can cause a severe drop in blood pressure. Death from respiratory depression may follow. Naloxone is a specific antidote for a Vicodin overdose.

NOTES

Introduction

1. C. Madren, "Investigating the Future of Forensics," American Association for the Advancement of Science, February 26, 2013, https://www.aaas.org/investigating-future-forensics.
2. "Exploring the History of Forensic Science through the Ages," Incognito Forensic Foundation, https://ifflab.org/history-of-forensic-science/.
3. N. Sheldon, "The Earliest Recorded Autopsy in History Was Performed on This Roman Emperor," https://historycollection.co/julius-caesar-complicit-death-re-examining-earliest-autopsy-history/; W. Shakespeare, *The Tragedy of Julius Caesar*, http://shakespeare.mit.edu/julius_caesar/full.html.
4. Ci. Song, *Xi Yuan Ji Lu Annotation,* Chinese ed. (Shanghai Ancient Books Publishing House, April 1, 2014), https://www.amazon.com/Xi-Yuan-Ji-Annotation-Chinese/dp/7532571866; SR. Dillon, "Chemistry & Crime—A Brief History," Florida State University, Department of Chemistry and Biochemistry, https://www.chem.fsu.

edu/chemlab/chm1020c/01-1.php.

5. See note 2, above.

6. "Edmond Locard," The Forensic Library, http://aboutforensics. co.uk/edmond-locard/.

7. "Classification of Fingerprints: Henry System," https://www. livingston.org/cms/lib9/NJ01000562/Centricity/Domain/781/ Henry%20System%20of%20Classification%2014.pdf.

8. See notes 2 and 6, above.

9. EJ. Wagner, "The French Connection of Sherlock Holmes," February 25, 2011, https://ejdissectingroom.wordpress.com/2011/02/25/the-french-connection-of-sherlock-holmes/; See note 6, above.

10. "Locard's Exchange Principle," Forensic Handbook, August 12, 2012, https://www.forensichandbook.com/locards-exchange-principle/.

11. I. Cobain, "Killer Breakthrough—the Day DNA Evidence First Nailed a Murderer," The Guardian, June 7, 2016, https://www. theguardian.com/uk-news/2016/jun/07/killer-dna-evidence-genetic -profiling-criminal-investigation.

12. T. Radeska, "James Marsh Was a British Chemist Who Invented the Marsh Test for Detecting Arsenic and Tracing the Poison in the Body," The Vintage News, January 9, 2017, https://www. thevintagenews.com/2017/01/09/james-marsh-was-a-british-chemist-who-invented-the-marsh-test-for-detecting-arsenic-and-tracing-the-poison-in-the-body/.

13. JB. West, "Carl Wilhelm Scheele, the Discoverer of Oxygen, and a Very Productive Chemist," Am J Physiol Lung Cell Mol Physiol 307:L811-L816 (2014); See note 6, above.

14. See note 2, above.

15. See note 4, above.

16. See note 2, above.

17. See note 4, above.

18. "Karl Landsteiner Biographical," The Nobel Prize," https://www. nobelprize.org/prizes/medicine/1930/landsteiner/biographical/.

19. B. Levine, *Principles of Forensic Toxicology*, (AACC Press, 2nd ed., 2003), https://books.google.co.uk/

books?hl=en&lr=&id=k7BInEQ-iqgC&oi=fnd&
pg=PR7&dq=forensic+toxicology+drugs&ots=2
DNu-DGWIO&sig=HPAFBSFmHIxmubJRpJQ_
DpLCOq4#v=onepage&q=forensic%20toxicology%20
drugs&f=false; "Forensic Toxicology Primer," National Institute
of Standards and Technology, March 2017, https://www.nist.gov/
system/files/documents/2017/04/04/osac_ftoxprimer_mar2017_
final.pdf.

20. See note 2, above.

21. "A Simplified Guide to Toxicology," http://www.
forensicsciencesimplified.org/tox/Toxicology.pdf; OH. Drummer,
"Forensic Toxicology," EXS 100:579–603 (2010); See note 19, above.

22. MC. Yarema and CE. Becker, "Key Concepts in Postmortem Drug
Redistribution," Clin Toxicol 43(4):235–241 (2005).

23. "Physicians' Handbook on Medical Certification of Death," Centers
for Disease Control and Prevention, National Center for Health
Statistics, Department of Health and Human Services, 2003, https://
www.cdc.gov/nchs/data/misc/hb_cod.pdf.

24. "Daubert v. Merrell Dow Pharmaceuticals, Inc., JUSTIA US
Supreme Court. 509 U.S. 579 (1993)," https://supreme.justia.com/
cases/federal/us/509/579/.

25. "Frye v. United States, 293 F. 1013 D.C. Cir. (1923)," https://casetext.
com/case/frye-v-united-states-7.

1. Errol Flynn

1. "Errol Flynn (1909–1959)," Hollywood's Golden Age, http://www.
hollywoodsgoldenage.com/actors/flynn.html.

2. "Errol Flynn Biography," https://www.imdb.com/name/
nm0001224/bio.

3. J. Miller, "Errol Flynn's Illicit Romance With a 15-Year-Old, as
Remembered by The Last of Robin Hood," Vanity Fair, September
7, 2013, https://www.vanityfair.com/hollywood/2013/09/
errol-flynn-toronto-film-festival.

4. See note 2, above.

5. "The History of Metropolitan Vancouver," http://www.vancouverhistory.ca/archives_flynn.htm.

6. "Report of Inquiry as to Cause of Death of Errol Leslie Flynn," http://www.autopsyfiles.org/reports/Celebs/flynn,%20errol_report.pdf.

7. E. Lazarus, "Glen McDonald: Vancouver's Colorful Coroner," January 19, 2019, https://evelazarus.com/glen-mcdonald-vancouvers-colourful-coroner/; "The History of The Coroner's Court, Part 2: The Brilliant, Whiskey-Loving Coroner," Vancouver Police Museum, February 7, 2019, https://vancouverpolicemuseum.ca/the-brilliant-whiskey-loving-coroner/.

8. See note 6, above.

9. M. Daugherty and T. Byler, "Genital Wart and Human Papillomavirus Prevalence in Men in the United States from Penile Swabs: Results from National Health and Nutrition Examination Surveys," Sex Transm Dis. 45(6):412–416 (2018); See note 6, above.

10. See note 2, above.

11. See note 6, above.

12. "Cirrhosis," https://medical-dictionary.thefreedictionary.com/portal+cirrhosis; See note 6, above.

13. See note 6, above.

14. See note 2, above.

15. See note 6, above.

16. RC. Baselt, "Meperidine," (*Disposition of Toxic Drugs and Chemicals in Man*, Biomedical Publications, 10th ed., pp 656–659, Foster City, CA, 2014); See note 6, above.

17. See note 6, above.

18. GA. Keller, MC. Villa Etchegoyen, et al., "Meperidine-Induced QTc-Interval Prolongation: Prevalence, Risk Factors, and Correlation to Plasma Drug and Metabolite Concentrations," Int J Clin Pharmacol Ther. 55(3):275–285 (2017); MK. Song, EJ. Bae, et al., "QT Prolongation and Life Threatening Ventricular Tachycardia in a Patient Injected With Intravenous Meperidine (Demerol®)," Korean Circ J. 41(6):342–345 (2011); M. Behzadi, S. Joukar, et al., "Opioids

and Cardiac Arrhythmia: A Literature Review," Medical Principles and Practice 27:401–414 (2018).

19. "DBL™ Pethidine Hydrochloride Injection BP 50 mg/ml," New Zealand Data Sheet, https://www.medsafe.govt.nz/profs/Datasheet/d/dblPethidineinj.pdf.

20. See note 2, above.

21. See note 1, above.

22. See note 2, above.

23. See note 1, above.

24. B. Leach, "Gone With the Wind Star Confirms One of Hollywood's Most Talked-About Romances," The Telegraph, June 17, 2009, https://www.telegraph.co.uk/news/celebritynews/5557364/Gone-With-The-Wind-star-confirms-one-of-Hollywoods-most-talked-about-romances.html.

25. See note 1, above.

26. See note 2, above.

27. See note 1, above.

28. See note 2, above.

2.   Marilyn Monroe

1. S. Doll, "Marilyn Monroe's Final Years," https://entertainment.howstuffworks.com/marilyn-monroe-final-years.htm.

2. H. Hertel and D. Neff, "From the Archives: Marilyn Monroe Dies: Pills Blamed," Los Angeles Times, August 6, 1962, http://www.latimes.com/local/obituaries/archives/la-me-marilyn-monroe-19620806-story.html.

3. "Marilyn Monroe Biography," A&E Television Networks, original published date April 2, 2014, last update August 14, 2018, https://www.biography.com/people/marilyn-monroe-9412123.

4. See note 2, above.

5. H. Markel, "Marilyn Monroe and The Prescription Drugs That Killed Her," PBS News Hour, August 5, 2016, https://www.pbs.org/newshour/health/marilyn-monroe-and-the-prescription-drugs-that-killed-her.

6. "Was Marilyn Monroe Murdered?" http://dyingwords.net/tag/chloral-hydrate/#sthash.b7M1q22f.dpbs.

7. E. Pak, "Marilyn Monroe's Happy Birthday, Mr. President Turns 50," Biography, May 17, 2012, https://www.biography.com/news/marilyn-monroes-happy-birthday-mr-president-turns-50-20829307.

8. "Autopsy Report—Marilyn Monroe," August 27, 1962, Office of the Los Angeles County Coroner, http://www.autopsyfiles.org/reports/Celebs/monroe,%20marilyn_report.pdf.

9. J. Preston, "Dr. Thomas Noguchi: LA Coroner Confidential," The Telegraph, September 10, 2009, https://www.telegraph.co.uk/culture/film/6126892/Dr-Thomas-Noguchi-LA-coroner-confidential.html.

10. See note 8, above.

11. See note 2, above.

12. See note 8, above.

13. See note 1, above.

14. RC. Baselt, "Pentobarbital," (*Disposition of Toxic Drugs and Chemicals in Man*, 10th ed., pp 1575-1577, Biomedical Publications, Seal Beach, California); See note 8, above.

15. See note 8, above.

16. RC. Baselt and RH. Cravey, "A Compendium of Therapeutic and Toxic Concentration of Toxicologically Significant Drugs in Human Biofluids," J. Anal. Tox. 1:81–103 (1977); "Chloral Hydrate," International Programme on Chemical Safety (INCHEM), https://www.who.int/ipcs/publications/cicad/en/cicad25.pdf?ua=1.

17. See note 8, above.

18. See note 1, above.

19. See note 8, above.

20. "A Bizarre Press Conference about the Death of Marilyn Monroe - Dr. Theodore Curphey August 1962," https://www.youtube.com/watch?v=b-3a6pWt43I&t=435s; See note 8, above.

21. D. Mallia, "How Did Marilyn Monroe Die?" History News Network, Columbian College of Arts & Sciences, The George Washington University, January 16, 2012, https://historynewsnetwork.org/article/144427.

22. See notes 1 and 2, above.

23. S. Doll, "Marilyn Monroe's Early Life," https://entertainment. howstuffworks.com/marilyn-monroe-early-life.htm; "Birth Record—Norma Jeane Mortenson."

24. S. Jackson, "Marilyn Monroe Remembered in 9 Ways," Biography, August 5, 2013, https://www.biography.com/news/marilyn-monroe-remembered-in-9-ways; See S. Doll, note 23, above.

25. See note 23, above.

26. S. Kattler, "Marilyn Monroe: Fascinating Facts about the Real Woman behind the Legend," Biography, August 3, 2017, https://www.biography.com/news/marilyn-monroe-biography-facts.

27. See note 23, above.

28. See note 26, above.

29. See note 23, above.

30. S. Doll, "Marilyn Monroe's Later Career," https://entertainment. howstuffworks.com/marilyn-monroe-later-career.htm.

31. S. Doll, "Marilyn Monroe's Early Career," https://entertainment. howstuffworks.com/marilyn-monroe-early-career.htm.

32. See S. Jackson, note 24, above; See note 30, above.

33. See note 3, above; See S. Jackson, note 24, above.

34. See S. Doll, note 1, above; See notes 3 and 30, above.

35. See notes 3 and 30, above.

36. See notes 1 and 3, above.

37. See note 1, above.

38. See notes, 1, 7, and 26, above.

39. See note 7, above; See S. Jackson, note 24, above.

40. See note 7, above.

41. D. Kreps, "Marilyn Monroe's 'Happy Birthday, Mr. President' Dress Sells for $4.8 Million," Rolling Stone, November 19, 2016, https://www.rollingstone.com/culture/culture-news/marilyn-monroes-happy-birthday-mr-president-dress-sells-for-4-8-million-113128/.

42. See notes 1 and 3, above.

43. See notes 1 and 31, above.

44. See note 26, above.

45. "Marilyn Monroe - The Last Interview," https://www.youtube.com/watch?v=WrbgHj0bAL4; See note 26, above.

46. See note 26, above.

47. See note 24, above.

48. See note 30, above.

49. L. Banner, *Marilyn: The Passion and the Paradox*, (pp 196-197, Bloomsbury USA, New York, NY, July 17, 2012.)

50. See note 1, above.

51. See note 30, above.

52. "Marilyn Monroe Biography," https://www.imdb.com/name/nm0000054/bio; "Songfacts, Candle in the Wind by Elton John," https://www.songfacts.com/facts/elton-john/candle-in-the-wind; J. Draper, "Who's Who on the Beatles' 'Sgt. Pepper Lonely Hearts Club Band' Album Cover," May 26, 2017, https://www.udiscovermusic.com/stories/whos-who-on-the-beatles-sgt-peppers-lonely-hearts-club-band-album-cover/.

3. *Jimi Hendrix*

1. "Monika Dannemann Biography," https://www.thefamouspeople.com/profiles/monika-dannemann-11927.php.

2. "Hendrix Inquest Inconclusive," Rolling Stone, October 29, 1970, https://www.rollingstone.com/music/music-news/hendrix-inquest-inconclusive-186643/; "Open Verdict Given in Hendrix's Death," The New York Times, September 29, 1970, https://www.nytimes.com/1970/09/29/archives/open-verdict-given-in-hendrixs-death.html.

3. R. Crossan, "Hear My Train a Comin' - The Final Days of Jimi Hendrix, Luxury London," https://luxurylondon.co.uk/culture/entertainment/jimi-hendrix-biography-final-days; See note 2, above.

4. See note 2, above.

5. See notes 2 and 3, above.

6. "1970: Rock legend Hendrix Dies After Party," BBC News, September 18, 1970, http://news.bbc.co.uk/onthisday/hi/dates/

stories/september/18/newsid_3528000/3528692.stm

7. See note 2, above.

8. "Robert Donald Teare," https://peoplepill.com/people/donald-teare/.

9. See note 2, above.

10. "Jimi Hendrix: 1942–1970," Rolling Stone, October 15, 1970, https://www.rollingstone.com/music/music-news/jimi-hendrix-1942-1970-93969/.

11. See note 2, above.

12. "Death Certificate—Jimi Hendrix," http://www.autopsyfiles.org/reports/deathcert/hendrix,%20jimi_dc.pdf; See note 2, above.

13. See note 2, above.

14. M. Torres and M. Digiovanna, "Tyler Skaggs' Autopsy: Fentanyl, Oxycodone and Alcohol Led to Death by Choking on Vomit," Los Angeles Times, August 30, 2019, https://www.latimes.com/sports/angels/story/2019-08-30/tyler-skaggs-autopsy-report-fentanyl-oxycodone-alcohol-angels-rusty-hardin.

15. K. Davies, "Police Reopen Investigation of Jimi Hendrix's Death," AP News, December 11, 1993, https://apnews.com/476a8dad6757ecc42fe1b25d47c6e023.

16. J. Bennetto, "Hendrix Girl Backs Inquiry," The Independent, December 12, 1993, https://www.independent.co.uk/news/uk/new-hendrix-inquest-rejected-1427871.html.

17. "British Official Rejects New Inquest into Jimi Hendrix' Death," UPI, March 9, 1994, https://www.upi.com/Archives/1994/03/09/British-official-rejects-new-inquest-into-Jimi-Hendrix-death/3101763189200/; "New Hendrix Inquest Rejected," The Independent, March 9, 1994, https://www.independent.co.uk.news/uk/new-hendrix-inquest-rejected-1427871.html.

18. "Jimi Hendrix Biography," A&E Networks, original published date April 2, 2014, last updated November 12, 2019, https://www.biography.com/musician/jimi-hendrix.

19. "Jimi Hendrix Biography," https://www.imdb.com/name/nm0001342/bio; See note 6, above.

20. See note 10, above.

21. "Jimi Hendrix Biography," https://www.jimihendrix.com/biography.
22. See note 14, above.
23. See note 21, above.
24. See notes 18 and 21, above.
25. See note 21, above.
26. See note 18, above.
27. See notes 18 and 19, above.
28. See note 19, above.
29. "Café Wha? History," https://cafewha.com/affiliates. cfm?searchurl=history; See note 19, above.
30. See note 19, above.
31. See notes 19 and 21, above.
32. See note 21, above.
33. See notes 19 and 21, above.
34. See note 10, above.
35. See note 12, above.
36. See note 10, above.
37. See note 19, above.
38. See notes 18 and 19, above.
39. See note 19, above.
40. See note 3, above.
41. See note 19, above.
42. See note 10, above.
43. "Jimi Hendrix, In His Own Words: 'I dig Strauss and Wagner—Those Cats are Good'," The Guardian, December 7, 2013, https://www.theguardian.com/music/2013/dec/08/ jimi-hendrix-in-his-own-words.
44. See note 3, above.
45. See note 10, above.
46. See note 17, above.
47. See note 43, above.

4. Janis Joplin

1. "Highland Gardens Hotel. Our History," https://www. highlandgardenshotel.com/pages/our-history.html#; "Janis Joplin's Hotel Room," https://www.atlasobscura.com/places/ janis-joplins-hotel-room.

2. "Janis Joplin Biography," Rock & Roll Hall of Fame, https://www. rockhall.com/inductees/janis-joplin; "Goodbye, Janis Joplin," Rolling Stone, October 29, 1970, https://www.rollingstone.com/ music/music-news/goodbye-janis-joplin-68526/.

3. F. Mastropolo, "The Day Janis Joplin Died," October 4, 2015, https://ultimateclassicrock.com/janis-joplin-death/; P. Valdes-Dapena, "Janis Joplin's 1964 Porsche Sells for $1.76 Million," CNN, December 11, 2015, https://money-cnn.com/2015/12/10/luxury/ janis-joplin-porsche-auction/index.html; See note 2, above.

4. JD. Nash, "What Happened to Janis Joplin's Porsche?" January 19, 2018, https://www.americanbluescene.com/janis-joplins-porsche-1/; See P. Valdes-Dapena, note 3, above.

5. "Autopsy Report—Janis Joplin," http://www.autopsyfiles.org/ reports/Celebs/joplin,%20janis_report.pdf.

6. "Janis Joplin Biography," A&E Television Networks, original published date April 2, 2014, last updated August 2, 2019, https:// www.biography.com/musician/janis-joplin.

7. G. Gent, "Death of Janis Joplin Attributed to Accidental Heroin Overdose," The New York Times, October 6, 1970, https://archive. nytimes.com/www.nytimes.com/books/99/05/02/specials/joplin-obit2.html?module=inline; See note 5, above.

8. "Transcripts: The People of the State of California vs. Robert Kenneth Beausoleil," November 14, 1960.

9. "Grand Jury Transcripts: The People of the State of California vs. Charles Manson, Charles Watson, aka Charles Montgomery; Susan Atkins, aka Sadie Mae Glutz; Linda Kasabian, Patricia Krenwinkel and Leslie Sanston," December 8, 1969.

10. DE. Kneeland, "Manson Trial Is Told Mrs. LaBianca Was Stabbed

41 Times," The New York Times, August 29, 1970, https://www.nytimes.com/1970/08/29/archives/manson-trial-is-told-mrs-labianca-was-stabbed-41-times.html.

11. See note 5, above.

12. S. Dam-Larsen, M. Franzmann, et al., "Long Term Prognosis of Fatty Liver: Risk of Chronic Liver Disease and Death," Gut 53:750–755 (2004); M. Goldberg and CM. Thompson, "Acute Fatty Metamorphosis of the Liver," Ann Intern Med 55(3):416–432 (1961); See note 5, above.

13. "Woodstock—16/08/1969—Janis Joplin," https://www.youtube.com/watch?v=Lz7x5pMdN0c.

14. AW. Jones, "Postmortem Toxicology Findings from Medico Legal Investigations of Drug Related Deaths among the Rich and Famous," Toxicol Anal Clin 29:298–308 (2017).

15. "Janis Joplin—Ball & Chain—Monterey Pop," https://www.youtube.com/watch?v=X1zFnyEe3nE; RC. Baselt, "Heroin," (*Disposition of Toxic Drugs and Chemicals in Man*, 10th ed., pp 992-996, Biomedical Publications, Seal Beach, California, 2014).

16. See note 5, above.

17. "Janis Joplin Biography," https://www.imdb.com/name/nm0429767/bio; GG. Gaar, "Janis Joplin. American Singer," Britannica, https://www.britannica.com/biography/Janis-Joplin; "Janis Joplin Interview," https://www.youtube.com/watch?v=BOTEDnQ4Fvk; M. Dostis, "Looking Back on the Life of Janis Joplin 45 Years After Her Early Death," New York Daily News," October 4, 2015, https://www.nydailynews.com/entertainment/remembering-life-janis-joplin-35-years-death-article-1.2383613; J. Doyle, "Joplin's Shooting Star," December 7, 2009, https://www.pophistorydig.com/topics/janis-joplin-1966-1970/.

18. A. Vincent, "Janis Joplin: Why She Still Has a Piece of Our Heart," The Telegraph, January 19, 2016, https://www.telegraph.co.uk/music/artists/janis-joplin-why-she-still-has-a-piece-of-our-heart/; See note 17, above.

19. See note 17, above.

20. See note 2, above; See J. Doyle, note 17, above.

21. See note 17, above.

22. See notes 13 and 17, above.

23. See note 17, above.

24. See note 2, above.

25. "Heroin," National Institute of Drug Abuse, November 2019, https://www.drugabuse.gov/publications/drugfacts/heroin.

5.   Cass Elliot

1. M. Kielty, "45 Years ago: Cass Elliot's Mysterious Death Ends a Promising New Chapter," July 29, 2019, https://ultimateclassicrock.com/45-years-ago-cass-elliots-mysterious-death-ends-a-promising-new-chapter/.

2. "'Mama Cass' Elliot Dead," Rolling Stone, August 29, 1974, https://www.rollingstone.com/music/music-news/mama-cass-elliot-dead-47050/; See note 1, above.

3. "The Official Cass Elliot Website," http://www.casselliot.com/biography.htm; "Obituary: Professor Keith Simpson," https://www.tandfonline.com/doi/abs/10.3109/174530585009156004?journalCode=ijau19.

4. "Death Certificate—Ellen Naomi Cohen (Cass Elliot)," https://findadeath.com/mama-cass-elliot/.

5. "Cass Elliot Biography," https://www.imdb.com/name/nm0254177/bio.

6. DB. Green, "This Day in Jewish History—Singer Cass Elliot Dies," Haaretz, July 29, 2014, https://www.haaretz.com/jewish/.premium-this-day-singer-cass-elliot-dies-1.5257187; See note 3, above.

7. See note 1, above.

8. See note 6, above.

9. "Mama Cass Biography," A&E Television Networks, original published date April 2, 2014, last updated July 11, 2019, https://www.biography.com/musician/mama-cass; See note 5, above.

10. "Cass Elliot, Pop Singer, Dies; Star of the Mamas and Papas,"

The New York Times, July 30, 1974, https://www.nytimes/
com/1974/07/30/archives/cass-elliot-pop-singer-dies-star-of-the-
mamas-and-papas-a-hearty.html; See note 9, above.

[11] See note 5, above.

[12] See notes 5 and 10, above.

[13] See notes 6 and 10, above.

[14] See notes 1 and 10, above.

[15] See note 5, above.

[16] "Dream A Little Dream: Just A Catchin' Fire," http://www.
dennydoherty.com/dream/dream11.html.

[17] See note 5, above.

[18] See note 16, above.

[19] See note 5, above.

[20] "Mama Cass in Training for Night Club Re-Entry,"
Ocala Star Banner, December 15, 1972, htttps://news.
google.com/newspapers?nid=1356&dat= 19721215&id=AGdRA
AAAIBAJ&sjid=CwYEAAAAIBAJ&pg=5061,3404963.

[21] See note 5, above.

[22] PS. Taback, "Mama Cass Elliot," Jewish Women's
Archive, https://jwa.org/encyclopedia/article/elliot-
mama-cass\.

[23] See note 5, above.

[24] See note 1, above.

[25] See note 2, above.

[26] See note 5, above.

[27] "Annie Nightingale Profile," https://www.bbc.co.uk/programmes/
profiles/3MKXvnKJm1f1gJCgNKk48w4/annie-nightingale-profile.

[28] S. Kenchaiah, JC. Evans, et al., "Obesity and the Risk of Heart
Failure," N Engl J Med 247:305–313 (2002); IA. Ebong, DC. Goff,
et al., "Mechanisms of Heart Failure in Obesity," Obes Res Clin
Pract 8(6):e540-e548 (2014); C. Wong and TH. Marwick, "Obesity
Cardiomyopathy: Pathogenesis and Pathophysiology," Nature Clin
Prac Cardiovascular Med 4:436–554 (2007).

[29] MA. Albert, "Obesity Cardiomyopathy: Pathophysiology and

Evolution of the Clinical Syndrome," Am J Med Sci 321(4):225–236 (2001).

30. See note 2, above.

6.   *Elvis Presley*

1. "Elvis Presley Biography," https://www.imbdb.com/name/nm0000062/bio.
2. "Elvis: The Final Hours," https://www.youtube.com/watch?v=fDQZLyUU2D4&t=2847s.
3. G. Timmons, "The Death of the 'King': Remembering Elvis," original published date August 15, 2017, last updated July 17, 2019, https://www.biography.com/news/elvis-presley-death-40-years-later; F. Tennant, "Elvis Presley: Head Trauma, Autoimmunity, Pain, and Early Death," Practical Pain Management, 44–95 (2013).
4. H. Markel, "Elvis' Addiction was the Perfect Prescription for an Early Death," PBS News Hour, August 16, 2018, https://www.pbs.org/newshour/health/elvis-addiction-was-the-perfect-prescription-for-an-early-death; "Medical Examiner's Report on the Death of Elvis (1977)," Preslaw.info/medical-examiners-report-autopsy-on-the-death-of-elvis-presley.
5. See F. Tennant, note 3, above.
6. See notes 3 and 4, above.
7. See F. Tennant, note 3, above.
8. See G. Timmons, note 3, above.
9. See F. Tennant, note 3, above.
10. See H. Markel, note 4, above.
11. "Elvis Autopsy," www.king-elvis-presley.de/html/death-elvis-autopsy.html.
12. See note 4, above.
13. A. Higinbotham, "Doctor Feelgood," The Guardian, August 10, 2002, https://www.theguardian.com/theobserver/2002/aug/11/features.magazine27.
14. See F. Tennant, note 3, above; See note 13, above.

15. See F. Tennant, note 4, above.

16. See note 2, above.

17. See note 3, above.

18. See F. Tennant, note 3, above.

19. See note 1, above.

20. "Elvis Presley Biography," A&E Television Networks, original published date April 2, 2014, last updated December 16, 2019, https://www.biography.com/musician/elvis-presley.

21. See note 1, above.

22. "Elvis Presley Biography," Elvis Australia, January 1, 2016, https://biography.elvis.com/au.

23. See note 1, above.

24. G. Marcus, "Elvis Presley: The Ed Sullivan Shows," https://www.msopr.com/n-past-campaigns/elvis-presley-the-ed-sullivan-shows/.

25. See notes 2 and 24, above.

26. See note 22, above.

27. "Pat Boone Biography," https://patboone.com/media/bio/.

28. See note 13, above.

29. See note 1, above.

30. C. Kirchberg, *Elvis Presley, Richard Nixon, and the American Dream*, (McFarland, Jefferson, NC., 1999), https://archive.org/details/elvispresleyrich00kirc.

31. P. Guralnick, *Careless Love: The Unmaking of Elvis Presley*, (Back Bay Books, Boston, MA, 2000). https://archive.org/details/isbn_9780316332972.

32. See notes 1 and 31, above.

33. A. Greene, "Flashback: Elvis Presley's 'Aloha from Hawaii' Marks His Final Truly Great Moment," Rolling Stone, July 31, 2018, https://www.rollingstone.com/music/music-news/flashback-elvis-presleys-aloha-from-hawaii-marks-his-final-truly-great-moment-705310/.

34. See notes 1 and 13, above.

35. See note 27, above.

36. See G. Timmons, note 3, above.

37. See note 13, above.

38. See G. Timmons, note 3, above.

39. See note 1, above.

40. See note 24, above.

41. See note 1, above.

42. "Priscilla Presley talks about Elvis meeting The Beatles," September 6, 2015, https://priscilla.elvispresley.com.au/priscilla-presley-talks-about-elvis-meeting-the-beatles.shtml.

43. P. Windsor, "Elvis Presley—Still 'The King' 42 Years after His Death," Forbes, August 14, 2019, https://www.forbes.com/sites/pamwindsor/2019/08/14/elvis-preslcystill-the-king-41-years-after-his-death/#49df3aca5845.

44. See note 22, above.

45. See note 42, above.

46. See note 43, above.

47. Z. O'Malley Greenburg, "The Top-Earning Dead Celebrities of 2019," Forbes, October 20, 2019, https://www.forbes.com/sites/zackomalleygreenburg/2019/10/30/the-top-earning-dead-celebrities-of-2019/#77849e344e53.

48. "There are 84,000 Elvis Presley Impersonators in the US, According to the IRS. Other than Las Vegas and Memphis, Where do they tend to Live?" https://www.quora.com/There-are-84-000-Elvis-Presley-impersonators-in-the-US-according-to-the-IRS-Other-than-Las-Vegas-and-Memphis-where-do-they-tend-to-live.

49. See note 43, above.

7. Natalie Wood

1. "Natalie Wood Biography," A&E Television Networks, original published date April 2, 2014, last updated May 1, 2020, https://www.biography.com/actor/natalie-wood.

2. "Catalina Island," https://www.visitcatalinaisland.com/about-the-island/; M. Puente, "Natalie Wood's 'Suspicious' Death: What you Need to Know About this Hollywood Mystery," USA Today, February 1, 2018, https://www.usatoday.com/story/life/2018/02/01/

natalie-wood-who-she-how-she-died-and-what-you-need-know/1086573001/; S. Kashner, "Natalie Wood's Fatal Voyage," Vanity Fair, March 2000, https://www.vanityfair.com/news/2000/03/natalie-wood-s-fatal-voyage; N. Bitette, "Revisiting the Night of Natalie Wood's Tragic Death," New York Daily News, February 1, 2018, https://www.nydailynews.com/entertainment/gossip/revisiting-night-natalie-wood-tragic-death-article-1.3793099; R. Bergara, S. Madej, et al., "What Happened to Famous Actress Natalie Wood?" BuzzFeed, September 8, 2017, https://www.buzzfeed.com/ryanbergara/the-mysterious-death-of-famous-actress-natalie-wood.

3. P. Crespo, "What Really Happened the Night Natalie Wood Died," HuffPost, November 18, 2015, updated December 6, 2017, https://www.huffpost.com/entry/what-really-happened-the_b_8594972; "Autopsy Report—Natalie Wagner (also known as Natalie Wood)," County of Los Angeles, Chief Medical Examiner-Coroner, December 5, 1981, http://www.autopsyfiles.org/reports/Celebs/wood,%20natalie_report.pdf; A. Zimmerman, "Inside the Mysterious Death of Natalie Wood," The Daily Beast, February 1, 2018, https://www.thedailybeast.com/inside-the-mysterious-death-of-natalie-wood-4; See S. Kashner, note 2, above; See N. Bitette, note 2, above.

4. See P. Crespo, note 3, above; See "Autopsy Report—Natalie Wagner," note 3, above.

5. See "Autopsy Report—Natalie Wagner," note 3, above.

6. See R. Bergara, S. Madej, et al., note 2, above; See P. Crespo, note 3, above; See "Autopsy Report—Natalie Wagner," note 3, above.

7. See P. Crespo, note 3, above.

8. See P. Crespo, note 3 above; See "Autopsy Report—Natalie Wagner," note 3, above.

9. See "Autopsy Report—Natalie Wagner," note 3, above.

10. See notes 2 and 3, above.

11. See P. Crespo, note 3, above.

12. See "Autopsy Report—Natalie Wagner," note 3, above.

13. "Natalie Wood Biography," https://www.imdb.com/name/nm0000081/bi; "Natalie Wood. Documentary," https://www.

youtube.com/watch?v=qwNqpmB-4Fs.

14. See "Autopsy Report—Natalie Wagner," note 3, above.

15. "Thomas Noguchi Biography," https://www.who2.com/bio/thomas-noguchi/; "Dr. Thomas Noguchi, the 'Coroner to the Stars' Demoted," UPI Archives, April 29, 1982, https://www.upi.com/Archives/1982/04/29/Dr-Thomas-Noguchi-the-coroner-to-the-stars-demoted/7106388900800/.

16. See "Autopsy Report—Natalie Wagner," note 3, above.

17. MD. Pérez-Cárceles, S. del Pozo, et al., "Serum Biochemical Markers in Drowning: Diagnostic Efficacy of Strontium and Other Trace Elements," Frensic Sci Int. 214(1–3):159–166, 2012; BL. Zhu, K. Ishida, et al., "Possible Postmortem Serum Markers for Differentiation between Fresh-, Saltwater Drowning and Acute Cardiac Death: A Preliminary Investigation," Leg Med (Tokyo). Suppl. 1:S298-S301, 2003.

18. See "Autopsy Report—Natalie Wagner," note 3, above.

19. "Understanding the Dangers of Alcohol Overdose," National Institute of Alcohol Abuse and Alcoholism. https://pubs.niaaa.nih.gov/publications/AlcoholOverdoseFactsheet/Overdosefact.htm; "Your Body at Different Levels of Blood Alcohol Concentration," https://www.alcohol.org/effects/blood-alcohol-concentration/.

20. M. Balsamo, "Natalie Wood's Drowning Now Considered a 'Suspicious Death'," Chicago Tribune, February 1, 2018, https://www.chicagotribune.com/entertainment/ct-natalie-wood-drowning-new-interest-20180201-story.html; J. Shamsian, "There's a New Twist in Natalie Wood's Unsolved Murder Case—Here's Everything You Need to Know," MSN Entertainment. July 24, 2018, https://www.msn.com/en-us/movies/celebrity/theres-a-new-twist-in-natalie-woods-unsolved-murder-case-%E2%80%94-heres-everything-you-need-to-know/ar-BBKZGW4; E. Jensen, "Natalie Wood's Death: Here's Why the Decades-Old Case is Making Headlines Again," USA Today. July 23, 2018, https://www.usatoday.com/story/life/entertainthis/2018/07/23/natalie-wood-death-fatal-voyage-podcast/817930002/; "Lakshmanan Sathyavagiswaran,

MD," https://www.ficsonline.org/m/pages.cfm?pageid=3940.

21. See "Autopsy Report—Natalie Wagner," note 3, above.

22. See R. Bergara, S. Madej, et al., note 2; See "Autopsy Report—Natalie Wagner," note 3, above.

23. M. Kaminsky, "Could 'Fatal Voyage' Podcast Lead to Arrest in 1981 Death of Natalie Wood?" Forbes, August 3, 2018, https://www.forbes.com/sites/michellefabio/2018/08/03/could-fatal-voyage-podcast-lead-to-arrest-in-1981-death-of-natalie-wood/#544720fe31d9; "Natalie Wood's Death Certificate Amended," BBC News, August 22, 2012, https://www.bbc.com/news/entertainment-arts-19341547; See "Autopsy Report—Natalie Wagner," note 3, above.

24. See "Autopsy Report—Natalie Wagner," note 3, above.

25. See P. Crespo, note 3, above.

26. "Natalie Wood (1938–1981)," Hollywood's Golden Age, http://www.hollywoodsgoldenage.com/actors/natalie-wood.html; D. Di Mambro, "Natalie Wood: A Tribute," http://www.classichollywoodbios.com/nataliewood.htm; "Natalie Wood Biography," September 14, 2017. https://www.thefamouspeople.com/profiles/natalie-wood-4020.php.

27. S. Gonzalez and L. Respers France, "Investigators say Robert Wagner's Story on Natalie Wood's Death Doesn't 'Add Up'," CNN, February 6, 2018, https://www.cnn.com/2018/02/05/entertainment/natalie-wood/index.html; A. Jenkins, "Natalie Wood's Death Has Been Ruled Suspicious. Here's what to Know about the Actor's Mysterious Drowning," Time, February 2, 2018, http://time.com/5131096/natalie-wood-robert-wagner/; See note 26, above.

28. See notes 13 and 26, above.

29. See notes 26 and 27, above.

30. See note 26, above.

31. See note 1, above.

32. See note 13, above.

33. See notes 26 and 27, above.

34. See S. Gonzalez and L. Respers France, note 27, above.

35. See notes 26 and 27, above.

36. See note 13, above.

37. C. Goffard, K. Mather, et al., "L.A. County Coroner Changes Natalie Wood's Cause of Death," Los Angeles Times, January 14, 2013, https://www.latimes.com/local/la-xpm-2013-jan-14-la-me-01-14-natalie-wood-20130115-story.html; See M. Balsamo, note 20, above.

38. P. Sherwell, "Natalie Wood was too 'Terrified' of Water to Try to Leave Robert Wagner on Yacht by Dinghy," The Telegraph, November 19, 2011, https://www.telegraph.co.uk/news/celebritynews/8901179/Natalie-Wood-was-too-terrified-of-water-to-try-to-leave-Robert-Wagner-on-yacht-by-dinghy.html.

39. P. Saperstein, "Natalie Wood Death: 'We're Closer to Understanding What Happened,' Say Investigators," Variety, February 5, 2018, https://variety.com/2018/film/news/natalie-wood-death-robert-wagner-lapd-1202687677/; M. Salam, "New Doubts in Natalie Wood's Death: 'I Don't Think She Got in the Water by herself,'" The New York Times, February 3, 2018, https://www.nytimes.com/2018/02/03/arts/natalie-wood-drowning-robert-wagner.html.

40. See J. Shamsian, note 20, above.

41. See J. Shamsian, note 20, above; See note 23, above.

42. See N. Bitette, note 2, above; See A. Zimmerman, note 3, above.

43. "Natalie Wood case: 'We're closer to Understanding What Happened! Detective Says," ABC News, February 6, 2018, https://www.abc13.com/entertainment/detectives-closer-to-understanding-natalie-wood-case-/3041953/; See "Autopsy Report—Natalie Wagner," note 3 above.

44. "Billy Joel - The Good Die Young with Lyrics," https://www.youtube.com/watch?v=zhjNm20XbXw.

8. John Belushi

1. "John Belushi Biography," http://belushi.com/bio.

2. "Autopsy Report—John Belushi," Department of Coroner, Los Angeles County, California, March 5, 1992, http://www.autopsyfiles.org/reports/Celebs/belushi,%20john_report.pdf; "John Belushi Biography," original published date April 2, 2014, last

updated October 8, 2019, https://www.biography.com/performer/john-belush*i*.

3. See "Autopsy Report—John Belushi," note 2, above.

4. C. Bertram, "The Final Days of John Belushi: What Led to His Sudden Death?" Biography, original published date May 20, 2019, last updated June 21, 2019, https://www.biography.com/news/john-belushi-death-final-days; See "Autopsy Report—John Belushi," note 2 above.

5. See "Autopsy Report—John Belushi," note 2, above.

6. See note 2, above.

7. See "Autopsy Report—John Belushi," note 2, above.

8. "Obituary: Dr. Ronald Kornblum, Former L.A. County Coroner," Mercury News, September 27, 2008, https://www.mercurynews.com/2008/09/27/obituary-dr-ronald-kornblum-former-l-a-county-coroner/.

9. See "Autopsy Report—John Belushi," note 2, above.

10. "John Belushi Biography," https://imdb.com/name/nm0000004/bio.

11. See notes 1 and 10, above.

12. H. Freeman, "The Tragic Legacy of John Belushi: 'He Could Have Done Anything.'" The Guardian, January 11, 2019, https://www.theguardian.com/film/2019/jan/11/tragic-legacy-john-belushi-actor-died-overdose.

13. See note 4, above.

9.   Karen Carpenter

1. "Autopsy Report—Karen Carpenter," http://www.autopsyfiles.org/reports/Celebs/carpenter,%20karen_report.pdf.

2. T. Eames, "The Tragic Story of Karen Carpenter, One of the Greatest Vocalists of All Time," original published date March 27, 2019, updated March 28, 2019, https://www.smoothradio.com/artists/carpenters/karen-carpenter-death-story-solo-album-husband/; See note 1, above.

3. See note 1, above.

4. "Carpenters Bio," www.richardandkarencarpenter.com/ biography-1.htm.

5. R. Schmidt, "Karen Carpenter's Tragic Story," The Guardian, October 23, 2010, https://www.theguardian.com/books/2010/oct/24/ karen-carpenter-anorexia-book-extract; See note 4, above.

6. See note 4, above.

7. See notes 2 and 4, above.

8. See note 5, above.

9. See notes 4 and 5, above.

10. See note 5, above.

11. See notes 4 and 5, above.

12. See note 5, above.

13. See notes 4 and 5, above.

14. See note 5, above.

15. MR. Sandar, A. Greway, et al., "Cardiovascular Impact of Eating Disorders in Adults: A Single Center Experience and Literature Review," https://www.ncbi.nlm.nih.gov/pmc/articles/PMC4590190/; J. Smythe, C. Colebourn, et al., "Cardiac Abnormalities Identified with Echocardiography in Anorexia Nervosa: Systematic Review and Meta-Analysis," Br J Psychiatry 6:1–10 (2020).

16. "Singer Karen Carpenter's Heart Stopped Because Of Irregularities in …," UPI Archives, March 11, 1983, https://www.upi.com/ Archives/1983/03/11/Singer-Karen-Carpenters-heart-stopped-because-of-irregularities-in/9152416206800/.

17. See note 1, above.

18. J. Samberg, "Remembering Karen Carpenter, 30 Years Later," National Public Radio, February 4, 2013, https://www.npr. org/2013/02/04/171080334/remembering-karen-carpenter-30-years-later; See note 2, above.

19. See note 4, above.

20. D. Tauriello, "What Do You Know About … Karen Carpenter?" Modern Drummer, 2013, https://www.moderndrummer.com/article/ december-2013-know-karen-carpenter/; See note 4, above.

21. See note 4, above.

22. See note 2, above.

23. WW. Gull, "V.—Anorexia Nervosa (Apepsia Hysterica, Anorexia Hysterica)," Obesity Res. 5(5):498–502 (1997), https://onlinelibrary. wiley.com/doi/abs/10.1002/j.1550-8528.1997.tb00677.x; C. Arnold, "Anorexia: You Don't Just Grow Out of It," The Guardian, March 29, 2016, https://www.theguardian.com/society/2016/mar/29/ anorexia-you-dont-just-grow-out-of-it.

24. "Anorexia Nervosa," National Eating Disorders Association, https://www.nationaleatingdisorders.org/learn/by-eating-disorder/ anorexia.

25. See note 5, above.

26. See note 16, above.

27. D. Wild, "Elton John: Sir Bitch Is Back," Rolling Stone, November 25, 2004, https://www.rollingstone.com/music/music-news/ elton-john-sir-bitch-is-back-240965/.

10. Sam Kinison

1. A. Wallace, "Friends Shocked by Violent Death of Mellower Kinison: Entertainer: The shock comedian was sobering up, associates say. A teen-ager is held in the collision," The Los Angeles Times, April 12, 1992, https://www.latimes.com/archives/la-xpm-1992-04-12- mn-456-story.html.

2. A. Srivatsa, "Sam Kinison's Cause of Death: How Did Sam Kinison Die?" December 20, 2017, https://www.earnthenecklace.com/sam- kinison-cause-of-death-accident-documentary/; See note 1, above.

3. "Autopsy Report—Samuel B. Kinison," http://www.autopsyfiles. org/reports/Celebs/kinison,%20sam_report.pdf; See note 1, above.

4. "Discover Needles," http://www.cityofneedles.com/Pages/ Government/City-Council.html; See note 3, above.

5. See "Autopsy Report—Samuel B. Kinison," note 3, above.

6. "Tranquilizers, Cocaine Found in Kinison's System," Los Angeles Times, May 29, 1992, https://www.latimes.com/archives/la-xpm- 1992-05-29-mn-346-story.html.

7. See A. Srivatsa, note 2, above; See note 4, above.

8. "Sam Kinison Biography," A&E Television Networks, original published date April 2, 2014, last updated April 18, 2019, https://www.biography.com/performer/sam-kinison; S. Palace, "The Scream of Sam Kinison—Religious Preacher Turned Rock Star Comedian," The Vintage News, December 17, 2018, https://www.thevintagenews.com/2018/12/17/sam-kinison/.

9. "Sam Kinison Candid Interview with Larry King," https://www.youtube.com/watch?v=HWxOMtZZrG8; "Sam Kinison @ The Joan Rivers Show," https://www.youtube.com/watch?v=L26pNwkWjN0; D. Jones, "Icon: Sam Kinison," GQ Magazine, April 20, 2012, https://www.gq-magazine.co.uk/article/sam-kinison-tribute-death-wild-thing-quotes-video ?v=KAQevjujhww.

10. "Rodney Dangerfield Biography," A&E Television Networks, original published date April 2, 2014, last updated July 18, 2019, https://www.biography.com/performer/rodney-dangerfield; See note 8, above.

11. See note 8, above.

12. See notes 9 and 10, above.

13. See note 8, above.

14. S. Holden, "Nine Comedians Appear on Dangerfield Special," The New York Times, August 2, 1985, https://www.nytimes.com/1985/08/02/arts/nine-comedians-appear-on-dangerfield-special.html.

15. D. Handelman, "The Devil and Sam Kinison," Rolling Stone, February 23, 1989, https://www.rollingstone.com/culture/culture-news/the-devil-and-sam-kinison-63844/.

16. "Sam Kinison First Appearance on Letterman," November 14, 1985, https://www.youtube.com/watch?v=m_VURr6jnWQ.

17. "Sam Kinison Biography," https://www.imdb.com/name/nm0455630/bio.

18. See note 8, above.

19. "Sam Kinison on Johnny Carson - May 24th, 1989," https://www.youtube.com/watch?v=7y6OukJ1G3I.

20. See note 8, above.

21. "Shock Comic Sam Kinison Killed in Head-on Car Crash," UPI Archives, April 11, 1992, https://www.upi.com/Archives/1992/04/11/Shock-comic-Sam-Kinison-killedin-head-on-car-crash/4355702964800/.

22. K. Jones, "Sam Kinison's Road to Self-Destruction," The Baltimore Sun, June 27, 1994, https://www.baltimoresun.com/news/bs-xpm-1994-06-27-1994178125-story.html.

23. A. McCartney, "Kinison Friend Says Comic Fathered Child," Washington Times, February 17, 2011, https://www.washingtontimes.com/news/2011/feb/17/kinison-friend-says-comic-fathered-child/.

24. Wenn, "Kinison Fathered Lovechild, Pal Says," Toronto Sun, February 19, 2011, http://www.torontosun.com/entertainment/celebrities/2011/02/19/17337136-wenn-story.html; "Sam Kinison's Secret Love Child: DNA Test Allegedly Prove a Friend's Daughter was Fathered by the Late Comic," The Daily Mail, February 18, 2011, https://www.dailymail.co.uk/news/article-1358387/Sam-Kinisons-secret-love-child-DNA-test-friends-daughter-fathered-late-comic.html.

25. See note 8, above.

26. See note 22, above.

27. See note 9, above.

28. See K. Jones, note 9, above.

29. See K. Jones, note 9, above; See note 25, above.

30. See note 9, above.

31. See note 25, above.

32. See note 1, above.

11. River Phoenix

1. "Biography of River Phoenix, Life, Death and Cause of Death," https://heightline.com/biography-river-phoenix-life-death-death/; "River Phoenix Biography," A&E Television Networks, original published date January 2, 2014, last updated January 14, 2020,

https://www.biography.com/actor/river-phoenix.

2. F. Wilkins, "The Untimely Death of River Phoenix," http://reelreviews.com/shorttakes/phoenix.htm; "Autopsy Report—River J. Phoenix," http://www.autopsyfiles.org/reports/Celebs/phoenix,%20river_report.pdf.

3. See notes 1 and 2, above.

4. See note 2, above.

5. See "Autopsy Report—River J. Phoenix," note 2, above.

6. See notes 1 and 2, above.

7. See note 1, above.

8. See "Autopsy Report—River J. Phoenix," note 2, above.

9. V. Kuklenski, "Coroner: Phoenix died of massive drug overdose," UPI Archives, November 12, 1993, https://www.upi.com/Archives/1993/11/12/Coroner-Phoenix-died-of-massive-drug-overdose/5534753080400/.

10. S. Mydans, "Death of River Phoenix is Linked to Use of Cocaine and Morphine," The New York Times, November 13, 1993, https://www.nytimes.com/1993/11/13/us/death-of-river-phoenix-is-linked-to-use-of-cocaine-and-morphine.html.

11. "Stand by Me," https://www.youtube.com/watch?v=WuxxjACRiNI.

12. "All in the Family," https://www.imdb.com/title/tt0066626/.

13. "Rob Reiner Biography," https://www.imdb.com/name/nm0001661/.

14. "Stand by Me. (1986)," https://www.imdb.com/title/tt0092005/; "River Phoenix Biography," https://www.imdb.com/name/nm0000203/.

15. See notes 1 and 14, above.

16. H. Freeman, "The untold story of River Phoenix, 25 years after his death," Irish Times, October 25, 2018, https://www.irishtimes.com/culture/film/the-untold-story-of-river-phoenix-25-years-after-his-death-1.3675342.

17. G. English, "This is what happened on the night River Phoenix died," October 26, 2018, https://www.msn.com/en-gb/entertainment/celebrity/this-is-what-happened-on-the-night-river-phoenix-died/ar-BBOV5X4.

18. M. Callahan, "River Phoenix's final hours," New York Post, September 22, 2013, https://nypost.com/2013/09/22/river-phoenixs-final-hours/.

19. See note 14, above.

20. See note 10, above.

21. H. Phoenix, "A Mother's Note on Her Son's Life and Death," Los Angeles Times, November 24, 1993, https://www.latimes.com/archives/la-xpm-1993-11-24-ca-60381-story.html.

22. See note 16, above.

12.   JonBenét Ramsey

1. "Wolf v. Ramsey, 253 F. Supp. 2d 1323 (N.D. Ga. 2003)," United States District Court for the Northern District of Georgia, Atlanta Division, March 31, 2003, https://law.justia.com/cases/federal/district-courts/FSupp2/253/1323/2567726/.

2. C. Brennan, "JonBenét Ramsey's Death a Tragic, Bizarre Case from the Start," The Daily Camera, January 27, 2013, https://www.dailycamera.com/2013/01/27/jonbenet-ramseys-death-a-tragic-bizarre-case-from-the-start/.

3. See note 1, above.

4. "JonBenét Ramsey," Crime Museum, https://www.crimemuseum.org/crime-library/cold-cases/jonbenet-ramsey/.

5. See note 1, above.

6. See notes 1 and 4, above.

7. See note 1, above.

8. See notes 1 and 4, above.

9. "Autopsy Report—JonBenét Ramsey," Office of the Boulder County Coroner, Boulder, Colorado, http://www.autopsyfiles.org/reports/Other/ramsey,%20jonbenet_report.pdf.

10. See note 1, above.

11. See note 9, above.

12. See note 1, above.

13. See note 9, above.

14. See note 1, above.

15. See note 9, above.

16. "JonBenét Ramsey Biography," https://www.imdb.com/name/nm2338600/bio; "Jon Benét Ramsey Biography," A&E Networks, original published date April 2, 2014, last updated December 13, 1999, https://www.biography.com/crime-figure/jonbenet-ramsey.

17. See notes 9 and 16, above.

18. See note 16, above.

19. See note 1, above.

20. See note 2, above.

21. See note 1, above.

22. See notes 1 and 2, above.

23. See note 1, above.

24. K. Auge, "JonBenét Ramsey," Denver Post, October 14, 1999, https://extra.denverpost.com/news/ram1014a.htm; C. Anderson, "Burke Ramsey not Suspect in Killing, DA's office," The Daily Camera, http://web.dailycaamera.com/extra/ramsey'1999/21arams.htm.

25. See note 1, above.

26. See note 1, above; See K. Auge, note 24, above.

27. "Ramsey Press Release," Boulder County Government, July 9, 2008, https://web.archive.org/web/20080801081500/http://www.bouldercounty.org/newsroom/templates/?a=1256&z=13; M.T. Lacy, "Letter to John Ramsey," Twentieth Judicial District, District Attorney's Office, July 9, 2008, https://wayback.archive-it.org/all/20081218174842/http://www.9news.com/pdfs/ramseyDA.pdf.

28. JJ. Maloney and P. O'Connor, "The Murder of JonBenét Ramsey," Crime Magazine, original published date May 7, 1999, last updated October 25, 2013, https://web.archive.org/web/20141129041656/http://www.crimemagazine.com/murder-jonben%C3%A9t-ramsey.

29. J. Brooke, "Bungled JonBenét Case Bursts a City's Majesty," The New York Times, December 5, 1997, https://www.nytimes.com/1997/12/05/us/bungled-jonbenet-case-bursts-a-city-s-majesty.html.

30. K. Wynne, "JonBenét Ramsey's Possible Killer May Have Confessed to Witnessing her Death in Letter From Prison,"

Newsweek, September 4, 2019, https://www.newsweek.com/ jonbenet-ramseys-possible-killer-may-have-confessed-witnessing-her-death-letters-prison-1457631; A. McDonell-Parry, "Pedophile Confesses to Killing JonBenét Ramsey in Letters to Friend," Rolling Stone, January 11, 2019, https://www.rollingstone.com/culture/ culture-news/jonbenet-ramsey-murder-gary-oliva-confession-letters-778025/; Z. Ferguson, "Where Is John Mark Karr, The Man Who Falsely Confessed to JonBenét Ramsey's Murder, & What Is He Doing Now?" The Bustle, March 26, 2015, https://www.bustle. com/articles/72098-where-is-john-mark-karr-the-man-who-falsely-confessed-to-jonbenet-ramseys-murder-what.

31. "JonBenét: DNA Rules out Parents," CBS News, December 16, 2004, https://www.cbsnews.com/news/jonbenet-dna-rules-out-parents/.

32. See note 4, above.

33. V. Miller, "Boulder Police Take Back Ramsey Case," Colorado Daily, February 2, 2009, https://web.archive.org/web/20150923205547/ http://www.coloradodaily.com/ci_13112748.

34. See MT. Lacy, note 27, above.

35. Y. Juris, "Who Is Mary Lacy? The JonBenét Ramsey District Attorney Issued an Important Apology," The Bustle, September 14, 2016, https://www.bustle.com/articles/183084-who-is-mary-lacy-the-jonbenet-ramsey-district-attorney-issued-an-important-apology; "Obituary Andrew "Lou" Smit. April 14, 1935 - August 11, 2010," https://www.dignitymemorial.com/obituaries/colorado-springs-co/andrew-smit-4345862; M. Brinlee, "Where Is Mark Beckner Now? The Former JonBenet Ramsey Police Chief Is Putting His Experience to Good Use," The Bustle, September 7, 2016, http:// www.bustle.com/articles/182291-where-is-mark-beckner-now-the-former-jonbenet-ramsey-police-chief-is-putting-his-experience-to.

36. See note 29, above.

13.   Anna Nicole Smith

1.   N. Finn, "The Weird, Wild and Tragically Short Life of Anna Nicole

Smith," November 28, 2018, https://www.eonline.com/news/896532/
the-weird-wild-and-tragically-short-life-of-anna-nicole-smith.

2. "Anna Nicole Smith Biography," Fox News, January 13, 2015,
    https://www.foxnews.com/story/anna-nicole-smith-biography.

3. H. Ryan, "Anna Nicole Smith's Last Days: Too Weak to Walk or Sit
    Up," Los Angeles Times, October 14, 2009, https://www.latimes.
    com/archives/la-xpm-2009-oct-14-me-anna-nicole14-story.html;
    L. Miller and B.L. Heldman, "Drugs, Feces and the Final Days of
    Anna Nicole Smith," October 13, 2009, https://www.eonline.com/
    news/148763/drugs-feces-and-the-final-days-of-anna-nicole-smith;
    M. Newman, "Cause of Anna Nicole Smith's Death Uncertain,"
    The New York Times, February 9, 2007, https://www.nytimes.
    com/2007/02/09/us/09cnd-smith.html; M. Sedensky, "Smith Died
    from Accidental Drug Overdose," AP News, March 26, 2007,
    https://web.archive.org/web/20070331213201/http://news.yahoo.
    com/s/ap/20070326/ap_on_en_tv/anna_nicole_smith.

4. J. Perper, "Background Information Pertaining to the Forensic
    Investigation into the Death of Anna Nicole Smith," March 2007,
    https://www.whiteplainspublicschools.org/cms/lib/NY01000029/
    Centricity/Domain/1128/anna%20nicole%20smith.pdf.

5. "Autopsy Report—Vickie Lynn Marshall," Broward County Medical
    Examiner, February 9, 2007, http://www.autopsyfiles.org/reports/
    Celebs/smith,%20anna%20nicole_report.pdf.

6. See note 4, above.

7. See notes 4 and 5, above.

8. See note 5, above.

9. See note 4, above.

10. See notes 4 and 5, above.

11. See note 4, above.

12. See note 5, above.

13. See note 4, above.

14. See notes 4 and 5, above.

15. See note 5, above.

16. See notes 4 and 5, above.

17. See note 4, above.

18. See notes 4 and 5, above.

19. "Anna Nicole Smith," https://www.thefamouspeople.com/profiles/anna-nicole-smith-3617.php; GG. Witch, "The Life of Anna Nicole Smith," https://reelrundown.com/celebrities/The-Life-of-Anna-Nicole-Smith; "Anna Nicole Smith Biography," A&E Television Networks, original published date April 2, 2014, last updated April 17, 2019, https://www.biography.com/people/anna-nicole-smith-183547; E. Stoddard and J. Rinaldi, "High School Remembers Anna Nicole—Barely," Reuters, February 9, 2007, https://web.archive.org/web/20070212044127/http://news.yahoo.com/s/nm/20070209/us_nm/annanicole_mexia_dc; *Anna Nicole Smith.* http://www.itsvery.net/anna-nicole-smith.html.

20. See note 1, above.

21. See E. Stoddard and J. Rinaldi, note 19, above.

22. See note 19, above.

23. "Dateline 20/20 ABC: Anna Nicole Smith: Beauty Lost," https://www.youtube.com/watch?v=RodM0JzhNK0.

24. "Final24 08 Anna Nicole Smith," https://www.youtube.com/watch?v=lpTTdPPpblM.

25. "Rare Anna Nicole Smith Interview Regis Philbin 1992 GUESS JEANS," https://www.youtube.com/watch?v=6C-u5J6oqP4.

26. "Anna Nicole Smith. Biography," https://www.imdb.com/name/nm0000645/bio; J. Molony, "Tragic tale of Anna Nicole, A Trailer-Trash Princess," The Independent, August 11, 2014, https://www.independent.ie/style/celebrity/celebrity-features/tragic-tale-of-anna-ncole-a-trailertrash-princess-30490758.html.

27. See notes 1 and 2, above.

28. See note 23, above.

29. See note 1, above.

30. M. Boardman, "Guess Founder Paul Marciano Talks Working with Naomi, Paris and Anna Nicole," Paper, July 18, 2017, http://www.papermag.com/paul-marciano-guess-anna-nicole-2456905932.html.

31. "Anna Nicole Smith Bio und Prozess," Berliner Zeitung,

August 5, 2010, https://www.bz-berlin.de/galerie-archiv/
anna-nicole-smith-bio-und-prozess.

32. See GG. Witch, note 19, above.

33. See notes 1 and 2, above.

34. "Anna Nicole Smith at the Billboard Awards," 2004, https://www.
youtube.com/watch?v=NzUU5J5E95c; J. Noveck, "What Drew
Us to Anna Nicole," Washington Post, February 8, 2007, http://
www.washingtonpost.com/wp-dyn/content/article/2007/02/08/
AR2007020801676_pf.html.

35. "Anna Nicole Oops on TV," https://www.youtube.com/
watch?v=sfBJtihEsGc.

36. "MTV Awards Australia 2005 - Anna Nicole Smith - Topless - 4
March 2005," https://www.youtube.com/watch?v=ciGmnaWvTTo

37. See note 26, above.

38. See note 2, above.

39. M. Memmott, "Supreme Court Rules against Anna Nicole Smith's
Estate," National Public Radio, June 23, 2011, https://www.
npr.org/sections/thetwo-way/2011/06/23/137366848/supreme-
court-rules-against-anna-nicole-smiths-estate; KP. Erb, "Judge
in Decades Old Anna Nicole Smith Case Announces He's Had
Enough," Forbes, January 30, 2017, https://www.forbes.com/sites/
kellyphillipserb/2017/01/30/judge-in-decades-old-anna-nicole-
smith-case-announces-hes-had-enough/#76b82c8833e9atch?v=ci
GmnaWvTTo.

40. See note 26, above.

41. P. Turnquest, "Birkhead is Father of Anna Nicole's Baby," Reuters.
April 10, 2007. https://www.reuters.com/article/us-annanicole/
birkhead-is-father-of-anna-nicoles-baby-idUSN1040771120070410

42. See note 26, above.

43. A. Goodnough and M. Fox, "Anna Nicole Smith Dies at 39,"
The New York Times, February 8, 2007, https://www.nytimes.
com/2007/02/08/arts/08cnd-smith.html.

44. See note 26, above.

45. See J. Noveck, note 34, above.

46. See note 1, above.

47. See H. Ryan, note 3 above; See L. Miller and BL. Heldman, note 3, above.

48. See note 19, above.

49. See M. Newman, note 3, above.

50. See note 26, above.

51. See J. Noveck, note 34, above.

14. Heath Ledger

1. J. Barron, "Heath Ledger, Actor, Is Found Dead at 28," The New York Times, January 23, 2008, https://www.nytimes.com/2008/01/23/ movies/23ledger.html; "Ledger's Death Caused by Accidental Overdose," CNN, February 2, 2008, https://www.cnn.com/2008/ SHOWBIZ/Movies/02/06/heath.ledger/; "Details Into the Death of Heath Ledger," original published date January 24, 2008, last updated June 30, 2008, https://www.wflx.com/story/7767445/ details-into-the-death-of-heath-ledger/.

2. "Heath Ledger Cause of Death," The City of New York, Department of Health & Mental Hygiene, February 6, 2008.

3. See note 1, above.

4. See note 2, above.

5. "Heath Ledger Biography," A&E Television Networks, original published date April 2, 2014, last updated August 27, 2019, https:// www.biography.com/actor/heath-ledger.

6. "Heath Ledge Biography," https://www.imdb.com/name/ nm0005132/bio; "Heath Ledger Dies of Accidental Prescription Drug Overdose," A&E Television Networks, original published date November 13, 2009, last updated July 27, 2019, https://www.history.com/this-day-in-history/ heath-ledger-dies-of-accidental-prescription-drug-overdose.

7. See note 1, above.

8. "Heath Ledger," https://www.tvguide.com/celebrities/heath-ledger/ credits/153347/.

9. See note 6, above.

10. K. Sessums, "We're Havin' a Heath Wave," Vanity Fair, January 23, 2008, https://www.vanityfair.com/news/2000/08/heath200008.

11. See note 6, above.

12. See note 1, above.

13. M. Betancourt, "I Am Heath Ledger Reveals the Struggle between the Actor and the Man," Esquire, May 17, 2017, https://www.esquire.com/entertainment/movies/a55102/heath-ledger-documentary/.

14. See note 10, above.

15. "Benzodiazepines and Opioids," National Institute on Drug Abuse, March 2018, https://www.drugabuse.gov/drugs-abuse/opioids/benzodiazepines-opioids.

16. N. Dasgupta and MJ. Funk, "Cohort Study of the Impact of High-Dose Opioid Analgesics on Overdose Mortality," Pain Med 17(1):85–98 (2016).

17. See note 15, above.

18. See note 1, above.

15.   Michael Jackson

1. C. Lee, and H. Ryan, "Michael Jackson's Last Rehearsal: Just Beaming with Gladness," Los Angeles Times, June 27, 2009, https://www.latimes.com/la-et-jackson-rehearsal27-2009jun27-story.html.

2. "A Timeline of Michael Jackson's Last Day," The Associated Press, June 20, 2010, https://www.newsday.com/entertainment/celebrities/a-timeline-of-michael-jackson-s-last-day-1.2041078.

3. "Autopsy Report—Michael Jackson," Department of Coroner, County of Los Angeles, August 19, 2009, http://www.autopsyfiles.org/reports/Celebs/jackson,%20michael_report.pdf.

4. RJ. Levy, "The Michael Jackson Autopsy: Insights Provided by a Forensic Anesthesiologist," J. Forensic Res. 2(8):1–7, 2011. https://www.omicsonline.org/peer-reviewed/the-michael-jackson-autopsy-insights-provided-by-a-forensic-anesthesiologist-2172.html; See note 3, above.

5. See note 3, above.

6. B. Barnes, "A Star Idolized and Haunted, Michael Jackson Dies at 50," The New York Times, June 25, 2009, https://www.nytimes.com/2009/06/26/arts/music/26jackson.html; See note 3, above.

7. See note 3, above.

8. "Conrad Murray Biography," A&E Networks, original published date April 2, 2014, last updated June 18, 2019, https://www.biography.com/personality/conrad-murray; "Dr. Conrad Murray: Trial Timeline," BBC News, November 30, 2011, https://bbc.com/news/entertainment-arts-15060651.

9. See note 3, above.

10. "The Jackson Family Biography," https://www.biography.com/people/groups/the-jackson-family; "Michael Jackson Biography," https://www.imdb.com/name/nm0001391/bio.

11. "Triumph & Tragedy: The Life of Michael Jackson," Rolling Stone India, August 25, 2009, http://rollingstoneindia.com/triumph-tragedy-the-life-of-michael-jackson.

12. "Michael Jackson Biography," A&E Television Networks, original published date April 2, 2014, last updated January 20, 2019, https://www.biography.com/people/michael-jackson-38211; "Michael Jackson Biography," https://www.biographyonline.net/music/michael-jackson.html.

13. See note 11, above.

14. See notes 10 and 12, above.

15. R. Vincent, "Michael Jackson," Britannica, February 1, 2019, https://www.britannica.com/print/article/ 298845.

16. See note 12, above.

17. See notes 12 and 15, above.

18. "Michael Jackson - Don't Stop 'Til You Get Enough (Official Video)," https://www.youtube.com/watch?v=yURRmWtbTbo.

19. "Michael Jackson Sweeps American Music Awards," The Daily News, January 17, 1984, https://news.google.com/newspapers?id=eQUbAAAAIBAJ&sjid=E0gEAAAAIBAJ&pg=5127,2841948.

20. "Michael Jackson: Heritage Award (proclaimed TRUE KING OF POP by Liz Taylor)," https://www.youtube.com/watch?v=d0vC_Ph7P9s.

21. B. McNulty, "Michael Jackson's music: the Solo Albums," The Telegraph, June 26, 2009, https://www.telegraph.co.uk/culture/music/michael-jackson/5652389/Michael-Jackson-music-the-solo-albums.html; T. Chan, "Michael Jackson Albums, Ranked," Spy, September 18, 2018, https://spy.com/2018/entertainment/books-music-movies/best-michael-jackson-albums-ranked-thriller-bad-off-the-wall-69171. "Motown 25: Yesterday, Today, Forever (1983)," https://www.imdb.com/title/tt0250595;

22. "Motown's 25th Anniversary Show. 1983," https://www.youtube.com/results?search_query=motown+25th+anniversary+full+show.

23. N. Murray, "When Michael moonwalked: Motown 25 Said Hi and Goodbye to Two Generations," September 29, 2014, https://www.avclub.com/when-michael-moonwalked-motown-25-said-hi-and-goodbye-1798272562.

24. See note 22, above.

25. R. Stone, "Inside Michael Jackson's Iconic First Moonwalk Onstage," Rolling Stone, October 5, 2015, https://www.rollingstone.com/music/music-news/inside-michael-jacksons-iconic-first-moonwalk-onstage-56650.

26. J. San, "35 Years Ago Today, Michael Jackson Moonwalked on TV for The First Time," Huffington Post, https://www.huffingtonpost.com/entry/35-years-ago-today-michael-jackson-moonwalked-on-tv-for-the-first-time_us_5afc8579e4b06a3fb50d1c7c.

27. See note 25, above.

28. See note 26, above.

29. S. Iyer, "Remembering the King of Pop: 10 signature Michael Jackson Dance Moves that Always Dazzled You," http://www.folomojo.com/remembering-the-king-of-pop-10-signature-michael-jackson-dance-moves-that-always-dazzled-you/.

30. L. Gotrich, "Michael Jackson's Gravity-Defying Lean Continues to Fascinate," National Public Radio, May 22, 2018, https://

www.npr.org/sections/therecord/2018/05/22/613306407/
michael-jacksons-gravity- defying-lean-continues-to-fascinate.

31. "Sammy Davis Jr. Biography," A&E Television Networks, original published date April 2, 2014, last updated April 27, 2017, https://www.biography.com/people/sammy-davis-jr-9268223.

32. "Leaving Neverland," 2019, https://www.imdb.com/title/tt9573980/.

16. Brittany Murphy

1. "Autopsy Report—Brittany Murphy-Monjack," Department of Coroner, County of Los Angeles, http://www.autopsyfiles.org/reports/Celebs/murphy,%20brittany_report.pdf.

2. "Dr. Lisa Scheinin, MD," https://www.healthgrades.com/physician/dr-lisa-scheinin-wb33h.

3. See note 1, above.

4. "Brittany Murphy Biography," A&E Television Networks, October 16, 2019, https://www.biography.com/actor/brittany-murphy; "Brittany Murphy Biography," https://www.imdb.com/name/nm0005261/bio.

5. A. Duke, "Coroner: No Indication Mold Killed Brittany Murphy or Simon Monjack," CNN, July 26, 2010, https://www.cnn.com/2010/SHOWBIZ/celebrity.news.gossip/07/26/murphy.monjack.mold/index.html.

6. AB. Block, "Shocking New Brittany Murphy Claim Says Toxic Mold May Have Killed Star," Hollywood Reporter, December 19, 2011, https://www.hollywoodreporter.com/thr-esq/brittany-murphy-death-mold-275478.

7. E. Lee, "Brittany Murphy's Cause of Death Could Be Reinvestigated," US Magazine, March 25, 2016, https://www.usmagazine.com/celebrity-news/news/brittany-murphys-cause-of-death-could-be-reinvestigated-w200271/.

8. 8. See note 4, above.

9. 9. "Brittany Murphy Died 10 Years Ago at 32: Inside Her Sudden Death That Still Confounds Hollywood,"

People, December 20, 2019, https://people.com/movies/brittany-murphy-died-10-years-ago-at-32-inside.

10. See note 1, above.

11. See note 7, above.

17. *Amy Winehouse*

1. M. Battersby, "'I don't want to die': Amy Winehouse's Words Just Hours Before her Death," The Independent, January 8, 2013, https://www.independent.co.uk/arts-entertainment/music/news/i-dont-want-to-die-amy-winehouses-words-just-hours-before-her-death-8442698.html; A. Topping, "Amy Winehouse Died of Alcohol Poisoning, Second Inquest Confirms," The Guardian, January 8, 2013, https://www.theguardian.com/music/2013/jan/08/amy-winehouse.

2. M. Turner, "Amy Winehouse Cause of Death Not Disclosed after Autopsy," The Hollywood Reporter, July 25, 2011, https://www.hollywoodreporter.com/news/amy-winehouse-cause-death-autopsy-214899-alcohol-poisoning-inquest; "Amy Winehouse Coroner's Inquest to be Reheard in London," BBC News, December 17, 2012, https://www.bbc.com/news/uk-england-london-20757135.

3. See note 1, above.

4. See M. Turner, note 2, above.

5. See note 2, above.

6. S. Hui, "Coroner: Amy Winehouse Died from Too Much Alcohol," Associated Press, October 26, 2011, http://archive.boston.com/ae/celebrity/articles/2011/10/26/inquest_to_hear_details_of_winehouses_final_hours/; "Coroner Reveals Amy Winehouse Death Cause," Associated Press, October 26, 2011, https://www.mysanantonio.com/news/article/Coroner-reveals-Amy-Winehouse-death-cause-2237186.php; See note 4, above.

7. 7. "Understanding the Dangers of Alcohol Overdose," National Institute on Alcohol Abuse and Alcoholism, https://www.niaaa.nih.gov/publications/brochures-and-fact-sheets/

understanding-dangers-of-alcohol-overdose; See note 6, above.

8. 8. See S. Hui, note 6, above.

9. 9. "Amy Winehouse Biography," https://www.imdb.com/name/nm1561881/bio-her-sudden-death-that-still-confounds-hollywood/.

10. "Resignation over Amy Winehouse Coroner Appointment," BBC News, December 12, 2012, https://www.bbc.com/news/uk-england-london-20695417.

11. "Amy Winehouse Inquest: Singer Drank Herself to Death," BBC News, January 8, 2013, https://www.bbc.com/news/uk-england-london-20944431.

12. A. Felton, "New Investigation Finds Excess Alcohol Killed Singer Amy Winehouse," CNN, January 8, 2013, https://www.cnn.com/2013/01/08/showbiz/uk-amy-winehouse-inquest/index.html.

13. See note 9, above.

14. "Amy Winehouse Biography," A&E Television Networks, original published date April 2, 2014, last updated January 16, 2019, https://www.biography.com/musician/amy-winehouse.

15. See note 9, above.

16. See note 14, above.

17. J. Eliscu, "Amy Winehouse's Death: A Troubled Star Gone Too Soon," Rolling Stone, July 24, 2011, https://www.rollingstone.com/music/music-news/amy-winehouses-death-a-troubled-star-gone-too-soon-188305/.

18. *Whitney Houston*

1. M. Seal M, "The Devils in the Diva," Vanity Fair, June 2012, https://www.vanityfair.com/hollywood/2012/06/whitney-houston-death-bathtub-drugs-rehab; "Autopsy Report—Whitney Houston," County of Los Angeles, Department of Coroner, February 12, 2012, http://www.autopsyfiles.org/reports/Celebs/houston,%20whitney_report.pdf.

2. S. Baltin, "Clive David Pre-Grammy Party Goes on in Memory of Whitney Houston," Rolling Stone, February 12, 2012, https://www.

334

rollingstone.com/movies/movie-news/clive-davis-pre-grammy-party-goes-on-in-memory-of-whitney-houston-115470/.

3. See note 1, above.

4. J. Pareles and A. Nagourney, "Whitney Houston, Pop Superstar, Dies at 48," The New York Times, February 11, 2012, https://www.nytimes.com/2012/02/12/arts/music/whitney-houston-dies.html.

5. P. Gallagher, "Whitney Houston Found Dead, Aged 48," The Guardian, February 11, 2012, https://www.theguardian.com/music/2012/feb/12/whitney-houston-dies-aged-48.

6. See "Autopsy Report—Whitney Houston," note 1, above.

7. A. Ballage, M. El Harti, et al., "Nasal Septum Perforation Due to Cocaine abuse," SAJ Case Rep 4:302–304 (2017); SA. Hardison, KK. Marcum, et al., "Severe Necrosis of the Palate and Nasal Septum Resulting from Intranasal Abuse of Acetaminophen," Ear Nose Throat J. 94:E40–42 (2015); See "Autopsy Report—Whitney Houston," note 1, above.

8. See "Autopsy Report—Whitney Houston," note 1, above.

9. A. Dasgupta, "Cocaethylene. Combined Alcohol and Drug Abuse," Alcohol Drugs, Genes, and the Clinical Laboratory, 2017, https://www.sciencedirect.com/topics/medicine-and-dentistry/cocaethylene.

10. See "Autopsy Report—Whitney Houston," note 1, above.

11. "Whitney Houston Biography," A&E Television Networks, original published date April 2, 2014, last updated January 16, 2019, https://www.biography.com/people/whitney-houston-9344818; "Whitney Houston Biography," https://www.imdb.com/name/nm0001365/bio?ref_=nm_ov_bio_sm; "Famous New Jerseyites," https://www.50states.com/bio/newjerse.htm.

12. "Transcript: Whitney Houston: 'I'm a Person Who Has Life,'" ABC News, February 13, 2012, https://abcnews.go.com/Entertainment/transcript-whitney-houston-im-person-life/story?id=15574357.

13. See note 11, above.

14. D. Shewey, "Whitney Houston," Rolling Stone, June 6, 1985, https://www.rollingstone.com/music/music-album-reviews/

whitney-houston-245970.

15. "Whitney Houston—Star Spangled Banner," https://www.youtube.com/watch?v=N_lCmBvYMRs.

16. D. Smith, "When Whitney Hit the High Note," ESPN, February 1, 2016, http://www.espn.com/espn/feature/story/_/id/14673003/the-story-whitney-houston-epic-national-anthem-performance-1991-super-bowl.

17. "Whitney Houston," People, https://people.com/archive/whitney-houston/.

18. "Houston W. Whitney: The Greatest Hits (DVD)," Sony BMG Music Entertainment, May 16, 2000, The Star Spangled Banner (Whitney Houston recording), https://en.wikipedia.org/wiki/The_Star_Spangled_Banner_(Whitney_Houston_recording).

19. R. O'Shea, "Pump Up Your Day with the Top 10 Sports Songs of All Time," Yahoo Sports, December 1, 2010, The Star Spangled Banner (Whitney Houston recording), https://en.wikipedia.org/wiki/The_Star_Spangled_Banner_(Whitney_Houston_recording); "The Star Spangled Banner (Whitney Houston recording)," https://en.wikipedia.org/wiki/The_Star_Spangled_Banner_(Whitney_Houston_recording).

20. MM. Evans, "'Whitney' Reflects on How the Singer's Iconic 1991 Super Bowl National Anthem Changed America in the Height of the Gulf War," Fox News, July 14, 1991, https://www.foxnews.com/entertainment/whitney-reflects-on-how-the-singers-iconic-1991-super-bowl-national-anthem-changed-america-in-the-height-of-the-gulf-war.

21. CJ. Lotz, "Why Dolly Parton "Will Always Love ..." That Song," Garden & Gun, February 12, 2018, https://gardenandgun.com/articles/dolly-parton-will-always-love-song.

22. A. Bucklow, "The Bodyguard: What You Never Knew about the Whitney Houston Movie," ABC News, https://www.news.com.au/entertainment/tv/flashback/the-bodyguard-what-you-never-knewabout-the-whitney-houston-movie/news-story/22fc997580e307a076adc903dcdabe15.

336

23. R. Ford, "Whitney Houston's 'The Bodyguard' to Re-Release in Theaters for One Night," Hollywood Reporter, March 15, 2012, https://www.hollywoodreporter.com/news/whitney-houston-bodyguard-theaters-kevin-costner-300684.

24. S. Rosenberg, "July 18, 1992: Whitney Houston Married Bobby Brown," https://www.mylifetime.com/she-did-that/july-18-1992-whitney-houston-married-bobby-brown; "Bobby Brown Charged with Battery," CNN Law Center, December 11, 2003, http://edition.cnn.com/2003/LAW/12/10/brown.charged/index.html; "Whitney & Bobby—Addicted to Love," September 2005, http://www.classicwhitney.com/interview/vibe_sep2005.htm.

25. L. McShane, "Whitney Houston Gets Bad Press," The Washington Post, April 6, 2000, http://www.washingtonpost.com/wp-srv/digest/ent3.htm.

26. A. Samuels, "Whitney Houston's Private Hell and Inevitable Death," Newsweek, April 30, 2012, https://www.newsweek.com/whitney-houstons-private-hell-and-inevitable-death-64115; A. Dansby, "Whitney Insider Tells of Drug Use, Failed Intervention," June 7, 2000, http://archive.li/7onCd.

27. S. Knolle, "Reports of Whitney Houston's Death Denied," ABC News, September 13, 2001, https://abcnews.go.com/Entertainment/reports-whitney-houstons-death-denied/story?id=102477.

28. See A. Samuels, note 26, above.

29. L. McNeil, "Inside Whitney Houston's Long Battle with Addiction: 'She Did Drugs to Escape the Pain,'" People, June 7, 2016, https://people.com/celebrity/whitney-houstons-long-battle-with-drug-addiction/.

30. "Fears for Whitney Houston Grow," Breaking News, November 9, 2001, https://www.breakingnews.ie/world/fears-for-whitney-houston-grow-23275.html; "Whitney Houston Admits to Drug Use in Diane Sawyer ABC News Interview," https://www.youtube.com/watch?v=8nzV5UL4CjA.

31. Wenn, "Houston Details Drug Use: 'We Laced Marijuana with Rock Cocaine.'" September 15, 2009, http://www.contactmusic.com/whitney-houston/news/

houston-details-drug-use-we-laced-marijuana-with-rock-cocaine_
1116018; "Whitney Houston Interview with Oprah Winfrey," https://
www.youtube.com/watch?v=KG42r7_2kOI.

32. See A. Dansby, note 26, above; See L. Mc Neil, note 29, above.

33. R. Kelly, "Cee Lo Rock Clive David Pre-Grammy Party; Whitney
Houston's Warwick Tribute Shaky," February 13, 20ll, https://
www.accessonline.com/articles/r-kelly-cee-lo-rock-clive-davis-pre-
grammy-party-whitney-houstons-warwick-tribute-shaky-96943.

34. "Whitney Houston. Biography," https://www.whitneyhouston.com/
biogrphy.

35. A. Light, "How a Director Uncovered Whitney Houston's Secret
Pain," The New York Times, July 13, 2018, https://www.nytimes.
com/2018/07/13/movies/whitney-houston-documentary.html.

36. "Whitney (2018)," https://www.imdb.com/title/tt5740866.

37. See note 35, above.

38. G. Palmer, "Whitney Houston Laid to Rest in New Jersey,"
Reuters, February 20, 2012, https://www.reuters.com/article/us-
whitneyhouston-burial/whitney-houston-laid-to-rest-in-new-jersey-
idUSTRE8II0M920120220.

39. "Whitney Houston Laid to Rest in Private Burial," Hollywood
Reporter, February 20, 2012, https://www.hollywoodreporter.com/
news/whitney-houston-death-funeral-292785.

40. A. Newcomb and S. Marikar, "Whitney Houston Funeral: Singer
Laid to Rest," ABC News, February 19, 2012, https://abcnews.
go.com/Entertainment/whitney-houston-funeral-singer-laid-rest/
story?id=15745349.

41. "This Day in Music. The Day The Music Died," http://www.
thisdayinmusic.com/pages/the_day_the_music_died.

42. T. Kenneally, "Whitney Houston Record Sales Soar in Days
after Death," Reuters, https://www.reuters.com/article/
idUS378724797120120215.

43. M. Puente, "Whitney Houston: Five Years after Her
Death, What's Happened?" USA Today, February 11, 2017,
https://www.usatoday.com/story/life/music/2017/02/10/

whitney-houston-five-years-after-her-death-whats-happened/97694288/.

44. See note 39, above.

45. See note 40, above.

46. See note 4, above.

19.   *Philip Seymour Hoffman*

1. D. Browne, "Philip Seymour Hoffman's Last Days," Rolling Stone, July 25, 2014, https://www.nme.com/news/philip-seymour-hoffman-mimi-odonnell-death-addiction-2171711; B. Weber, "Philip Seymour Hoffman, Actor of Depth, Dies at 46," The New York Times, February 3, 2014, https://www.nytimes.com/2014/02/03/movies/phili-seymour-hoffman-actor-dies-at-46-html; "Philip Seymour Hoffman Biography," https://www.imdb.com/name/nm0000450/bio.

2. R. Sanchez, "Coroner: Philip Seymour Hoffman died of acute drug mix intoxication," CNN, February 28, 2014, https://www.cnn.com/2014/02/28/showbiz/philip-seymour-hoffman-autopsy/index.html.

3. P. Reaney, "Philip Seymour Hoffman Dies of Accidental Overdose: Official," Reuters, February 28, 2014, https://www.reuters.com/article/us-philipseymourhoffman-autopsy/philip-seymour-hoffman-died-of-accidental-overdose-official-idUSBREA1R1X920140228.

4. See D. Browne, note 1, above.

5. "Philip Seymour Hoffman on Sobriety & Capote - 60 Minutes Full Interview (2006)," https://www.youtube.com/watch?v=-pLzxE0Rg5I; T. Vallance, "Philip Seymour Hoffman Obituary: Oscar-Winner for 'Capote' Acclaimed for an Indelible Succession of Haunting, Enigmatic Performances," The Independent, February 4, 2014, https://www.independent.co.uk/news/obituaries/philip-seymour-hoffman-oscar-winner-for-capote-acclaimed-for-an-indelible-succession-of-haunting-9105371.html.

6. R. Gilbey, "Philip Seymour Hoffman Obituary," The Guardian, February 3, 2014, https://www.theguardian.com/film/2014/feb/03/philip-seymour-hoffman; A. Green, "Mimi O'Donnell Reflects on the Loss of Philip Seymour Hoffman and the Devastation of Addiction," Vogue, December 13, 2017, https://www.vogue.com/article/philip-seymour-hoffman-mimi-odonnell-vogue-january-2018-issue.

7. See D. Browne, note 1, above.

8. See note 6, above.

9. LM. Britton, "Mimi O'Donnell, the Long-Term Partner of Late Actor Philip Seymour Hoffman, Has Penned an Emotional Tribute to the Star, Opening Up About His Death and Battle with Addiction," NME, December 14, 2017, https://www.nme.com/news/philip-seymour-hoffman-mimi-odonnell-death-addiction-2171711; E. Jensen, "Philip Seymour Hoffman's Partner Recounts How he Slid Back Into Drug Addiction," USA Today, December 14, 2017, https://www.usatoday.com/story/life/people/2017/12/14/mimi-odonnell-opens-up-ferocious-pain-philip-seymour-hoffmans-death/951063001/.

10. See A. Green, note 6, above.

11. See D. Browne, note 1, above.

12. See A. Green, note 6, above.

13. See notes 1, 2, and 3, above.

14. "Philip Seymour Hoffman Biography," A&E Networks, original published date April 1, 2014, last updated August 16, 2019, https://www.biography.com/actor/philip-seymour-hoffman.

15. L. Hirschberg, "A Higher Calling," The New York Times, December 19, 2008, https://www.nytimes.com/2008/12/21/magazine/21hoffman-t.html?pagewanted=all.

16. See note 1, above.

17. See note 15, above.

18. See notes 1 and 14, above.

19. See D. Browne, note 1, above.

20. See note 15, above.

21. See T. Vallance, note 5, above.

340

22. See note 14, above.

23. See B. Weber, note 1, above.

24. See note 13, above.

25. See B. Weber, note 1, above.

26. N. Murray, K. Phipps, et al., "The Dissolve Remembers Philip Seymour Hoffman," https://thedissolve.com/features/tribute/397-the-dissolve-remembers-philip-seymour-hoffman/.

27. See A. Green, note 6, above.

28. See note 1, above.

29. See A. Green, note 6, above.

30. See note 1, above.

31. See LM. Britton, note 9, above.

32. See A. Green, note 6, above.

20. Robin Williams

1. S. Youn, "Robin Williams: Autopsy Confirms Death by Suicide," Hollywood Reporter, November 7, 2014, https://www.hollywoodreporter.com/news/robin-williams-autopsy-confirms-death-746194.

2. "Autopsy Report—Robin McLaurin Williams," http://tmz.vo.llnwd.net/o28/newsdesk/tmz_documents/1107-robin-williams-coroners-report.pdf.

3. D. Itzkoff, "Inside the Final Days of Robin Williams," Vanity Fair, May 8, 2018, https://www.vanityfair.com/hollywood/2018/05/robin-williams-death-biography-dave-itzkoff-excerpt.

4. See note 2, above.

5. T. Walker, "Robin Williams Dead. Actor was Found Hanging in His Bedroom by His Personal Assistant, Police Say," The Independent, August 12, 2014, https://www.independent.co.uk/news/people/robin-williams-dead-police-say-actor-was-found-hanging-in-his-bedroom-by-personal-assistant-9665009.html.

6. See note 2, above.

7. "Joseph I. Cohen, MD," http://www.forensiconline.com/about.html.

8. See note 2, above.

9. P. Fimrite, E. Sernoffsky, et al., "Grim Details of Robin Williams' Death Released by Investigators," August 13, 2014, https://www.sfgate.com/bayarea/article/Investigators-Robin-Williams-hanged-himself.

10. See note 2, above.

11. "The Brain from Top to Bottom. Amyloid Plaques and Neurofibrillary Tangles," https://thebrain.mcgill.ca/flash/d/d_08/d_08_cl/d_08_cl_alz/d_08_cl_alz.html.

12. J. Sonne and MR. Beato, "Neuroanatomy, Substantia Nigra," Stat Pearls Publishing LLC, December 28, 2018, https://www.ncbi.nlm.nih.gov/books/NBK536995/.

13. See note 7, above.

14. "What is Lewy Body Dementia?" National Institute on Aging, NIH, https://www.nia.nih.gov/health/what-lewy-body-dementia#what -5683229.php.

15. See note 2, above.

16. NM. Smith, "Robin Williams' Widow: 'It was not Depression' that Killed Him," The Guardian, November 3, 2015, https://www.theguardian.com/film/2015/nov/03/robin-williams-disintegrating-before-suicide-widow-says.

17. G. Greengross, "Why Do Comedians Become Comedians?" Psychology Today, November 20, 2013, https://www.psychologytoday.com/us/blog/humor-sapiens/201311/why-do-comedians-become-comedians.

18. "Robin Williams Best American Actor and Comedian Biography Documentary Film," https://www.youtube.com/watch?v=1ufUJJUfEvo; "Robin Williams Biography," https://www.imdb.com/name/nm0000245/bio; "Robin Williams Biography," A&E Television Networks, original published date April 2, 2014, last updated August 1, 2019, https://www.biography.com/actor/robin-williams; "Robin Williams Biography," https://www.thefamouspeople.com/profiles/robin-mclaurim-williams-2733.php; "Robin Williams Biography: His Life was a Dark Comedy," Biographics, November 21, 2017, https://biographics.org/

robin-williams-biography-life-dark-comedy/.

19. S. Cahalan, "How Robin Williams was Being Torn Apart and Couldn't Fight back," New York Post, May 5, 2018, https://nypost. com/2018/05/05/how-an-incurable-brain-disease-haunted-robin-williams-final-days/.

20. "Robin Williams Interview on Donahue in 1989," https://www. youtube.com/watch?v=sQXg7Yxmb-Q; C. Bertram, "Robin Williams' Non-Stop Mind Brought Joy to Millions. But for Him, It Brought Endless Pain," May 6, 2019, https://www.biography.com/ news/robin-williams-mind-life-death.

21. See note 18, above.

22. M. Wojciechowski, "Na-Nu, Na-Nu! Remembering Mork & Mindy 40 Years Later," Parade, September 14, 2018, https://parade. com/424126/michelewojciechowski/na-nu-na-nu-remembering-mork-and-mindy/; "Mork & Mindy," https://www.imdb.com/title/ tt0077053/.

23. "Watch Mork and Mindy Season 1 Episode 1," https://www.youtube. com/watch?v=NLpzCNhA8vM.

24. See note 18, above.

25. R. Ebert, "Moscow on the Hudson," January 1, 1984, https://www. rogerebert.com/reviews/moscow-on-the-hudson-1984.

26. See note 18, above.

27. "The Cecil B. deMille Award," Golden Globes, https://www. goldenglobes.com/cecil-b-demille-award-0.

28. "Robin Williams' Heart Surgery: Road to Recovery," https://www.webmd.com/heart-disease/news/20090324/ robin-williams-heart-surgery-road-to-recovery#1.

29. See note 20, above.

30. See note 28, above.

31. See note 2, above.

32. D. Holahan, "Robin Williams Bio Revelations: Infidelity, Substance Abuse, Insecurity over Jim Carrey," USA Today, original published date May 7, 2018, last updated May 13, 2018, https://www.usatoday.com/story/life/books/2018/05/07/

robin-williams-bio-revelations-infidelity-depression-insecurity/587314002/.

33. See note 20, above.

34. See note 18, above.

35. SS. Williams, "The Terrorist inside My Husband's Brain," Neurology 87:1308–1311 (2016), https://n.neurology.org/content/87/13/1308.full.

36. See note 14, above.

37. See note 20, above.

38. See note 19, above.

39. See note 35, above.

40. H. Tohid, "Robin Williams' Suicide: A Case Study," Trends Psychiatry Psychother. 38(3):178–182 (2016), http://www.scielo.br/scielo.php?script=sci_arttext&pid=S2237-60892016000300178&lng=en&tlng=en.

41. See note 2, above.

21. Joan Rivers

1. S. Youn, "Joan Rivers' Fatal Surgery: What Went Wrong," Hollywood Reporter, November 11, 2014, https://www.hollywoodreporter.com/news/joan-rivers-fatal-surgery-what-748058.

2. M. Puente, "Year After Joan Rivers' Death, What Changed?" USA Today, September 4, 2015, https://www.usatoday.com/story/life/2015/09/04/one-year-anniversary-joan-rivers-death-what-happened-doctors-clinic/71649424/.

3. M. Santora, "Settlement Reached in Joan Rivers Malpractice Case," The New York Times, May 12, 2016, https://www.nytimes.com/2016/05/13/nyregion/settlement-reached-in-joan-rivers-malpractice-case.html.

4. "Joan Rivers Joked About her Death at her Final Comedy Show Hours before Heart Attack," ABC News, September 4, 2014, https://abc7ny.com/entertainment/photos-joan-rivers-final-stage-performance/286481/.

5. J. Bernstein, "For Joan Rivers' Doctor, Fame Delivers Its Bill," The New York Times, November 5, 2014, https://www.nytimes.com/2014/11/06/fashion/for-joan-rivers-doctor-Dr-Gwen-Korovin-fame-delivers-its-bill.html.

6. "Report on Clinic that treated Joan Rivers," Department of Health and Human Services, Centers for Medicare & Medicaid Services, September 5, 2014, http://s3.documentcloud.org/documents/1356659/report-on-clinic-that-treated-joan-rivers.pdf

7. G. Gavel, "Laryngospasm in Anesthesia," Continuing Education in Anesthesia Critical Care & Pain. 14(2), 2014; E. Hernandez-Cortez, "Update on the Management of Laryngospasm," J. of Anesthesia & Critical Care. 8(2):1–6 (2018.

8. See notes 1 and 6, above.

9. C. D'Auria and J. Smith, "Medical Examiner: Joan Rivers' Death 'Resulted From Predictable Complication,'" CBS Local, October 16, 2014, https://newyork.cbslocal.com/2014/10/16/medical-examiner-joan-rivers-death-resulted-from-predictable-complication/.

10. See note 6, above.

11. M. Farhan, MQ. Hoda, et al., "Prevention of Hypotension Associated with the Induction Dose of Propofol: A Randomized Controlled Trial Comparing Equipotent Doses of Phenylephrine and Ephedrine," J. Anesthesiol. Clin. Pharmacol. 31(4):526–530 (2015).

12. See G. Gavel, note 7, above.

13. See note 7, above.

14. See G. Gavel, note 7, above.

15. S. Rice, "Joan Rivers' Death Highlights Risks for seniors in Outpatient Surgery," Modern Health Care, September 13, 2014, https://www.modernhealthcare.com/article/20140913/MAGAZINE/309139963/joan-rivers-death-highlights-risks-for-seniors-in-outpatient-surgery.

16. L. Joszt, "Joan Rivers' Death Highlights Risks of Surgical Complications," MD Magazine, September 5, 2014, https://www.mdmag.com/medical-news/joan-rivers-death-highlights-risks-of-surgical-complications.

17. B. Ross and GA. Otis, "Joan Rivers' daughter, Melissa, Files Multimillion Dollar Lawsuit against Manhattan Clinic, Doctors Involved in Comedian's Fatal Surgery," New York Daily News, January 27, 2015, https://www.nydailynews.com/entertainment/gossip/joan-rivers-daughter-melissa-files-suit-mother-death-article-1.2092477.

18. See note 6, above.

19. See E. Hernandez-Cortez, note 7, above.

20. P. Reaney, "New York Clinic that Treated Comic Joan Rivers Sued Over her Death," Reuters, January 26, 2015, https://www.reuters.com/article/us-usa-rivers-lawsuit/new-york-clinic-that-treated-comic-joan-rivers-sued-over-her-death-idUSKBN0KZ2KO20150127; E. Yahr, "What Went Wrong with Joan Rivers' Last Medical Procedure: Lawsuit," Washington Post, January 28, 2015, https://www.washingtonpost.com/news/arts-and-entertainment/wp/2015/01/28/what-went-wrong-with-joan-riverss-last-medical-procedure-lawsuit/.

21. L. Le Vine, "Melissa Rivers Reaches Settlement in Medical-Malpractice Suit over Joan Rivers' Death," Vanity Fair, May 13, 2016, https://www.vanityfair.com/style/2016/05/melissa-rivers-settlement-medical-malpractice-suit-joan-rivers-death; "Melissa Rivers Settles Medical Malpractice Lawsuit Over Joan Rivers' Death," Hollywood Reporter, May 12, 2016, https://www.hollywoodreporter.com/news/joan-rivers-death-medical-malpractice-893559.

22. "Joan Rivers Biography," A&E Television Networks, original published date April 12, 2014, last updated June 17, 2019, https://www.biography.com/performer/joan-rivers.

23. RD. McFadden, "Joan Rivers, a Comic Stiletto Quick to Skewer, Is Dead at 81," The New York Times, September 4, 2014, https://www.nytimes.com/2014/09/05/arts/television/joan-rivers-dies.html.

24. See note 22, above.

25. B. Maranzani, "Inside Joan Rivers and Johnny Carson's Epic Falling Out," A&E Television Networks, June 20, 2019, https://www.biography.com/news/joan-rivers-johnny-carson-feud.

26. J. Rivers, "Joan Rivers: Why Johnny Carson "Never Ever Spoke to Me Again," Hollywood Reporter, December 6, 2012, https://www.hollywoodreporter.com/news/joan-rivers-why-johnny-carson-398088.

27. L. Bennetts, "Joan Rivers' Remarkable Rise to (and Devastating Fall from) Comedy's Highest Ranks," Vanity Fair, November 3, 2016, https://www.vanityfair.com/hollywood/2016/11/joan-rivers-last-girl-before-freeway-excerpt.

28. A. Heigl, "Joan Rivers, Johnny Carson & the Bumpy Road to Tonight," People, September 4, 2014, https://people.com/celebrity/joan-rivers-and-johnny-carsons-history-on-the-tonight-show/.

29. See note 26, above.

30. See note 28, above.

31. See note 23, above.

32. N. Finke, "Edgar Rosenberg: The Public Ending of a Private Life: Suicide of Rivers' Husband Came without a Warning," Los Angeles Times, August 20, 1987, https://www.latimes.com/archives/la-xpm-1987-08-20-vw-3767-story.html.

33. See note 27, above.

34. "Did Jackie Mason Give Ed Sullivan "the Finger" on National Television?" http://legendsrevealed.com/entertainment/2016/04/15/did-jackie-mason-give-ed-sullivan-the-finger-on-national-television/.

35. LA. Johnson, "Jackie Mason Skewers -- Well, Everything," South Florida Sun-Sentinel, February 24, 2001, https://www.sun-sentinel.com/news/fl-xpm-2001-02-24-0102230761-story.html.

36. See note 22, above.

37. See note 28, above.

38. "Joan Rivers Biography," https://www.imdb.com/name/nm0001672/bio.

39. See note 26, above.

40. V. Gay, "Was Johnny Carson Right, or was Joan Rivers Right? Let's Settle This!" Newsday, September 4, 2015, https://www.newsday.com/entertainment/tv/

joan-rivers-johnny-carson-feud-who-was-right-1.9233874.

41.	"Joan Rivers Visits Johnny Carson's Grave," https://www.youtube.com/watch?v=h8Mp_HnkWTk.

42.	See note 2, above.

43.	See note 38, above.

22.   *Prince*

1.	J. Coscarelli and SM. Eldred "Prince's Overdose Death Results in No Criminal Charges," The New York Times, April 19, 2018, https://www.nytimes.com/2018/04/19/arts/music/prince-death-investigation.html.

2.	"Carver County Attorney Mark Metz Announces no Criminal Charges Following the Prince Rogers Nelson Death Investigation," April 19, 2018, https://www.co.carver.mn.us/home/showdocument?id=13174.

3.	D. Chanen, "Prince Died from Accidental Overdose of Fentanyl," Star Tribune, June 3, 2016, http://www.startribune.com/prince-died-from-opioid-overdose/381663221/.

4.	See note 2, above.

5.	J. Eligon, SF. Kovaleski, et al., "Prince's Addiction and an Intervention Too Late," The New York Times, May 4, 2016, https://www.nytimes.com/2016/05/05/arts/music/friends-sought-help-for-princes-addiction-lawyer-says.html.

6.	J. Eligon and SF. Kovaleski, "Clues to the Mystery of Prince's Final Days," The New York Times, April 22, 2016, https://www.nytimes.com/2016/04/23/arts/music/prince-death-final-days.html.

7.	See note 5, above.

8.	See note 2, above.

9.	See note 6, above.

10.	S. Montemayer, "Carver County Closes Prince Death Investigation with no Criminal Charges," Star Tribune, April 20 2018, http://www.startribune.com/no-charges-in-prince-death-investigation/480252103/.

11.	See note 5, above.

12. See note 6, above.

13. "Watch Police News Conference on Prince's Death," PBS News Hour, https://www.youtube.com/watch?v=McmDZ8DNAGk.

14. See note 3, above.

15. See note 13, above.

16. See note 6, above.

17. See note 5, above.

18. See note 6, above.

19. "Prince Rogers Nelson," Midwest Medical Examiner's Office Press Release, https://www.co.carver.mn.us/home/showdocument?id=7465.

20. A. Forliti, "Experts: Prince Toxicology Report Shows Very High Drug Level," Associated Press, March 26, 2018, https://apnews.com/f80bf6952ecf4d02a675b9fac69d7dc6/Experts:-Prince-toxicology-report-shows-very-high-drug-level; RC. Baselt, "Fentanyl," (*Disposition of Toxic Drugs and Chemicals in Man*, Biomedical Publications, 10th ed., pp 846–849, Foster City, CA, 2014).

21. JE. Bromwich, "Prince Overdosed on Fentanyl. What Is It?" The New York Times, June 2, 2016, https://www.nytimes.com/2016/06/03/health/what-is-fentanyl.html.

22. See note 19, above.

23. "Attorney: No Criminal Charges in Prince's Death," CNN, https://www.youtube.com/watch?v=Co3Uh8_bKR8.

24. "Prince Biography," A&E Television Networks, original published date April 2, 2014, last updated October 22, 2019, https://www.biography.com/musician/prince.

25. "Prince Rogers Nelson's Entire 1999 CNN Interview (Larry King Live)," https://www.youtube.com/watch?v=m8mg7CxAYUM.

26. "Pop Prodigy: Teen Prince Debuted as Artist, Producer," Newsweek, April 26, 2016, https://www.newsweek.com/pop-prodigy-prince-artist-producer-teenager-452356.

27. "Prince Biography," https://www.imdb.com/name/nm0002239/bio.

28. S.T. Erlewine, "Dirty Mind," https://www.allmusic.com/album/dirty-mind-mw0000191363.

29. See note 24, above.

30. See note 25, above.

31. See note 27, above.

32. See note 24, above.

33. *Prince. The Beautiful Ones*, (Spiegel & Grau, New York, NY, October 29, 2019,) https://www.amazon.com/Beautiful-Ones-Prince/dp/0399589651/ref=tmm_hrd_swatch_0?_encoding=UTF8&qid=1579547413&sr=8-1.

34. See note 21, above.

35. See notes 3 and 5, above.

36. E. Levenson and H. Silverman, "No Criminal Charges in Prince's Death, Attorney Says," CNN, April 19, 2018, https://www.cnn.com/2018/04/19/us/prince-death-investigation/index.html.

37. See note 2, above.

38. "Fentanyl and Other Synthetic Opioids Drug Overdose Deaths," National Institute on Drug Abuse, https://www.drugabuse.gov/related-topics/trends-statistics/infographics/fentanyl-other-synthetic-opioids-drug-overdose-deaths.

39. See note 13, above.

40. See note 2, above.

41. See note 10, above.

23. *Carrie Fisher*

1. A. Bennett, "Details of Carrie Fisher's Cause of Death Revealed," Los Angeles Daily News, September 14, 2017, https://www.dailynews.com/2017/06/16/details-of-carrie-fishers-cause-of-death-revealed; S. Kelley and C. Littleton, "Carrie Fisher 'Star Wars' Actress and Writer Who Rocketed to Fame as Princess Leia, Dies at 60," Variety, December 27, 2016, https://variety.com/2016/film/news/carrie-fisher-dead-star-wars-princess-leia-dies-1201948744/.

2. J. Serna and R. Winton, "Carrie Fisher's Autopsy Reveals Cocktail of Drugs, Including Cocaine, Opiates, and Ecstasy," Los Angeles Times, June 19, 2017, https://www.latimes.com/

local/lanow/la-me-ln-carrie-fisher-autopsy-report-20170619-story.
html; "Autopsy Report—Carrie Fisher," County of Los Angeles,
Department of Coroner, January 3, 2017, http://www.autopsyfiles.
org/reports/Celebs/fisher,%20carrie_report.pdf.

3. R. Rubin, "Toxicology Tests Detect Variety of Drugs in Carrie
Fisher, but their Role in her Death Isn't Clear," Forbes, June 19, 2017,
https://www.forbes.com/sites/ritarubin/2017/06/19/toxicology-tests-
detect-variety-of-drugs-in-carrie-fisher-but-their-role-in-her-death-
isnt-clear/#7a538b8e1489.

4. See "Autopsy Report—Carrie Fisher," note 2, above.

5. "Carrie Fisher's Death: Explaining Cardiac Arrest vs. Heart
Attacks," USA Today, January 10, 2017, https://www.usatoday.
com/story/life/movies/2017/01/10/carrie-fishers-death-certificate-
confirms-heart-attack/96381322/; "Carrie Fisher's Death Certificate
Confirms Cardiac Arrest," CBS News, January 11, 2017, https://
www.cbsnews.com/news/carrie-fisher-death-certificate-confirms-
heart-attack; "Carrie Fisher: Hospital Confirms Heart Attack as
Cause of Death," Hollywood Reporter, January 9, 2017, https://
www.hollywoodreporter.com/carrie-fisher-cause-death-certificate-
confirms-heart-attack-963047; H. Ellis-Petersen, "Carrie Fisher had
Cocaine and Heroin in System When She Died, Coroner Finds," The
Guardian, June 19, 2017, https://www.theguardian.com/culture/2017/
jun/19/carrie-fisher-death-drugs-autopsy-coroner.

6. "Cardiac Arrest vs. Heart Attack," https://cpr.heart.org/AHAECC/
CPRAndECC/AboutCPRFirstAid/CardiacArrestvsHeartAttack/
UCM_473213_Cardiac-Arrest-vs-Heart-Attack.jsp; RF. Graham,
"Carrie Fisher 'Relapsed' Before European Tour that Ended in her
Death: Friend Claims Actress was 'High as a Kite' Over Thanksgiving
but Pressed Ahead with Ambitious Work Schedule that Saw her
Visit the UK Just Days Later," The Daily Mail, December 28, 2016,
https://www.dailymail.co.uk/news/article-4069614/Carrie-Fisher-
relapsed-European-tour-ended-death-Friend-claims-actress-high-
kite-Thanksgiving-pressed-ahead-ambitious-work-schedule.html.

7. See note 3, above.

8. See "Autopsy Report—Carrie Fisher," note 2, above.

9. "Carrie Fisher Biography," April 4, 2018, https://www. thefamouspeople.com/profiles/carrie-fisher-4686.php.

10. "When is an Autopsy Required in California?" https://ecobear.co/ crime-scene-cleaning/autopsy-required-california.

11. S. Abrams S, "LA County Names New Acting Coroner to Oversee Strapped Department," Los Angeles Daily News, January 19, 2017, updated August 29, 2017, https://www.dailynews.com/2017/01/19/ la-county-names-new-acting-coroner-to-oversee-strapped-department/.

12. M. Ishida, W. Gonoi, et al., "Common Postmortem Computed Tomography Findings Following Atraumatic Death: Differentiation between Normal Postmortem Changes and Pathologic Lesions," Korea J Radiol 16:798–809, 2015.

13. See note 2, above.

14. See J. Serna and R. Winton, note 2, above.

15. See J. Serna and R. Winton, note 2, above; See note 12, above.

16. See "Autopsy Report—Carrie Fisher," note 2, above.

17. "Physicians' Handbook on Medical Certification of Death," Centers for Disease Control and Prevention, National Center for Health Statistics, Department of Health and Human Services, 2003, https:// www.cdc.gov/nchs/data/misc/hb_cod.pdf.

18. See "Autopsy Report," note 2, above.

19. "Eddie Fisher Biography," A&E Television Networks, original published date April 2, 2014, last updated December 29, 2016, https://www.biography.com/people/eddie-fisher-604144; "Eddie Fisher Biography," https://www.imdb.com/name/nm0279472/bio.

20. W. Lerner, "Before Brad, Angelina, and Jennifer There was Elizabeth Taylor, Debbie Reynolds, and Eddie Fisher," July 5, 2018, https://www.yahoo.com/entertainment/brad-angelina-jennifer-elizabeth-taylor-debbie-reynolds-eddie-fisher-140049035.html; R. Bergan, "Debbie Reynolds Obituary," The Guardian, December 28, 2016, https://www.theguardian.com/film/2016/dec/29/ debbie-reynolds-obituary-singin-in-the-rain-actor.

21. See W. Lerner, note 20, above.

22. KM. Heussner, "Science of Beauty: What Made Elizabeth Taylor So Attractive?" ABC News, https://abcnews.go.com/Technology/elizabeth-taylor-science-great-beauty/story?id=13203775; "Debbie Reynolds Dead, Actress Once Known as "America's Sweetheart" was 84," CBS News, December 29, 2016, https://www.cbsnews.com/news/debbie-reynolds-once-known-as-americas-sweetheart-dead-at-84; "Debbie Reynolds Biography," https://www.imdb.com/name/nm0001666/bio.

23. "Carrie Fisher Biography," https://www.imdb.com/name/nm0000402/bio.

24. "Star Wars: Episode IV—A New Hope (1977)," https://www.imdb.com/title/tt0076759.

25. "Star Wars Databank: Mos Eisley Cantina," https://www.starwars.com/databank/mos-eisley-cantina.

26. "Carrie Fisher Biography," A&E Television Networks, original published date April 2, 2014, last updated January 30, 2018, https://www.biography.com/people/carrie-fisher-9542646.

27. See RF. Graham, note 6, above.

28. See note 23, above.

29. C. Fisher, *The Princess Diarist*, (Blue Rider Press, New York, NY, October 24, 2017); J. Miller, "Inside Carrie Fisher's Difficult Upbringing with Famous Parents," Vanity Fair, December 27, 2016, https://www.vanityfair.com/style/2016/12/carrie-fisher-parents-debbie-reynolds-eddie-hollywood.

30. "Bipolar Disorder," The National Institute of Mental Health, https://www.nimh.nih.gov/health/topics/bipolar-disorder/index.shtml; "BBC HARDtalk - Carrie Fisher - Actress (2000)," https://www.youtube.com/watch?v=rMUTSQPs2sA.

31. D. Itzkoff, "Carrie Fisher, Child of Hollywood and 'Star Wars' Royalty, Dies at 60," The New York Times, December 27, 2016, https://www.nytimes.com/2016/12/27/movies/carrie-fisher-dead-star-wars-princess-leia.html.

32. See RF. Graham, note 6, above.

[33.] See note 31, above.

[34.] See note 23, above.

[35.] See notes 23 and 26, above.

[36.] See C. Fisher, note 29, above.

24. *Conclusion*

[1.] I. Smith, "Psychostimulants and Artistic, Musical, and Literary Creativity," Int Rev Neurobiol. 120:301–326 (2015); L-SC. D'Angelo, G. Savulich, et al., "Lifestyle Use of Drugs by Healthy People for Enhancing Cognition, Creativity, Motivation and Pleasure," Br J Pharmacol 174:3257–3267 (2017); RM. Holm-Hadulla and A. Bertolino "Creativity, Alcohol and Drug Abuse: The Pop Icon Jim Morrison," Psychopathology 47(3): 167–173 (2014).

INDEX

dexamethasone, 189, 274
dextropropoxyphene, 274–75
diazepam, 63, 106, 113, 116, 140, 150, 158, 231, 275
DiMaggio, Joe, 30, 33
diphenhydramine, 140, 188, 192, 251, 275
diverticulae, 6
D-methamphetamine, 284
DNA analysis, xv, 111, 132, 146, 214
Doherty, Denny, 56–59
doxylamine, 150–51, 276
Doyle, Arthur Conan, xi
Doyle, Jack, 52
Dr. Nick, 70
drowning, 76, 78–79, 84, 191–92, 261, 313
Drug Enforcement Administration (DEA), 243, 245

E

Ecstasy, 184, 250, 276, 350
Elliot, Cass, 55–60, 102, 259–62
    autopsy of, 56
    cause and manner of death of, 57
    death of, 55–57, 60, 102, 259–62
    life and career of, 57–58
emetine cardiotoxicity, 98
eosinophils, 7, 173
ephedrine, 116, 276, 345
Erlewine, Stephen, 241

escitalopram, 135, 277
esophagogastroduodenoscopy (EGD), 223–25, 227–28
Etchingham, Kathy, 39
ethchlorvynol, 63, 277
ethinamate, 63, 277

F

fatty metamorphosis, 6, 19, 49, 62, 261
fatty myocardial degeneration, 56, 60
Federal Bureau of Investigation (FBI), xiv
fentanyl, 91, 239, 243–44, 278, 303, 348–50
fibroids, 191, 263
Fielder-Civil, Blake, 184
Filbin, Regis, 143
finasteride, 214, 278
fingerprint analysis, xiii–xiv
Finkle, Bryan S., 63
Fisher, Carrie, viii, 247–51, 253–57, 261, 350–53
    autopsy of, 249
    cause and manner of death of, 250–52
    death of, 247–52, 254, 256
    life and career of, 253, 255–56
Fisher, Eddie, 253, 352
Fitzgerald, Ella, 30–31
fluoxetine, 175, 251, 278

Printed in the United States
By Bookmasters